TO:

FROM:

DATE:

The ideas, concepts and opinions expressed in all Dexterity Publishing books and No Cheats Needed recipes are intended to be used for educational purposes only. The books and recipes are sold with the understanding that authors and publisher are not rendering medical advice of any kind, nor are the books or recipes intended to replace medical advice, nor to diagnose, prescribe or treat any disease, condition, illness or injury, nor make promises of weight loss.

It is imperative that before beginning any diet or exercise program, including any aspect of the No Cheats Needed program, you receive full medical clearance from a licensed physician.

Authors and publisher claim no responsibility to any person or entity for any liability, loss, or damage caused or alleged to be caused directly or indirectly as a result of the use, application or interpretation of the material in the books or recipes.

The Food and Drug Administration has not evaluated the statements contained on Nocheatsneeded.com, in any Dexterity Publishing books, or in the No Cheats Needed recipes.

Literary development and design: Koechel Peterson & Associates, Inc., Minneapolis, Minnesota.

Dexterity Publishing
P.O. Box 227357
Dallas, TX 75222

Printed in the United States of America

First Edition: September 2014
2 3 4 5 6 7 8 | 19 18 17 16 15 14

ISBN: 978-0-9908344-0-3

6 Weeks to a Healthier, Better You

No Cheats Needed

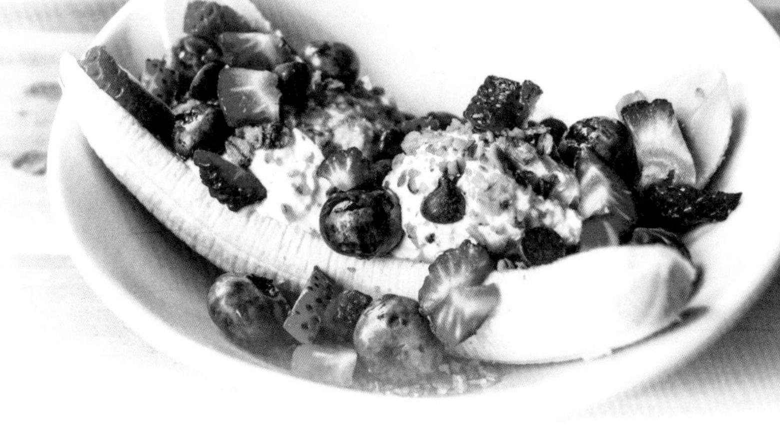

kevin curry

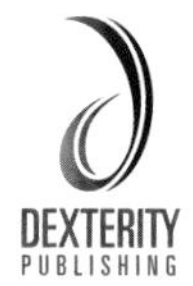

DEXTERITY
PUBLISHING

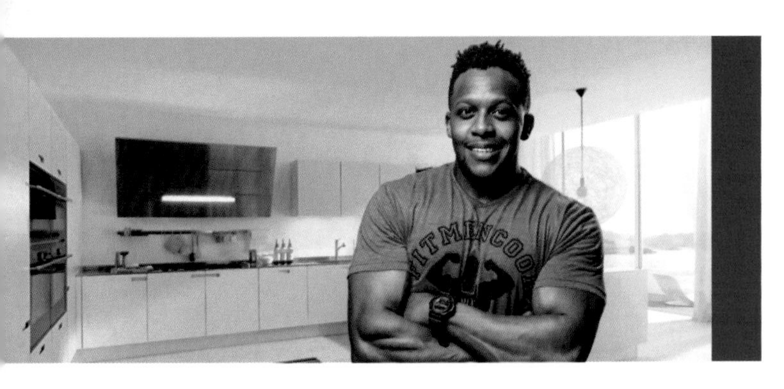

ABOUT KEVIN

In the Introduction, Kevin shares how seeing a photo of himself posted on Facebook led to a life-changing journey to becoming the founder of one of the most prolific social media followings in the world of nutrition. He is the self-taught cook behind @FitMenCook. Anyone who meets Kevin would describe him as a dynamic and inspiring personality, so it's hard to believe that underneath it all, Kevin also struggled with depression and food had evolved from a love to become an escape and, like for many others, a coping mechanism. Over time, he packed over 40 unhealthy pounds onto his frame that required a life makeover to overcome.

Kevin is a Texas and Harvard grad whose self-taught method has taken him from a behind-the-scenes career working in corporate America, to pursuing his passions full time in healthy food blogging. In 2012, he started blogging and sharing photos and content on Tumblr and Instagram. His initial Instagram page went from zero to over a quarter million followers in a matter of months. "I am not a chef. I studied nutrition and healthy ingredients and stepped into the kitchen to experiment with creating lean, fulfilling, macronutrient-dense meals for myself. *Eating healthy actually worked!"*

His mantra was cemented, and he has inspired countless thousands to lead healthier, more fulfilling lives. When not in the kitchen or gym, he can be found spending time with family and friends, incubating recipes for his cookbook series, working on start-up ideas with friends, rooting for the Texas Longhorns, and binging on Netflix.

. . . and if you were wondering, yes, Curry is his real last name. Enjoy!

Contents

INTRODUCTION

How did I transform my diet, my physique, and eventually, my career?

You wouldn't believe how many times I've been asked that question.

It all started with a Facebook photo.

After seeing a picture my friend uploaded, and kindly tagged, of me on Facebook, I knew I needed help. "How had I gained so much weight?" And more importantly, "Why didn't anyone say something to me?" However, regardless of how I got to the point of being considered obese, I was "comfortably" there and realized that I needed to make a change.

My struggle with food—*may be better characterized as an all-out war*—may sound familiar, so I'll spare you the details and give you the abbreviated version in just a few bullet points.

- *Guy gains weight.*
- *Guy hires a personal trainer for assistance with nutrition and exercise.*
- *Guy loses weight.*
- *Guy quickly becomes bored with the mundane diet of grilled chicken breast, steamed broccoli, and brown rice.*
- *Guy treats himself to his favorite food—Mexican food—and the robust flavors remind him all over again of why he became overweight. He lacked self-control when it came to food.*
- *Guy gains back the weight. . . .*
- *Guy becomes depressed and feels helpless.*

I was absolutely disappointed in myself and despised the reflection I saw in the mirror.

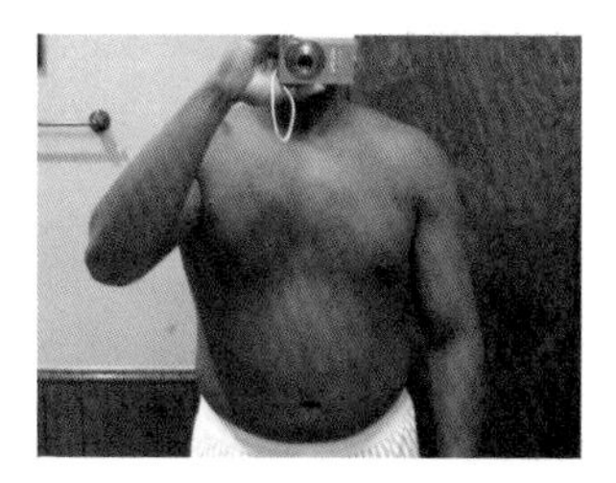

Picture from 2009. I was about 220 pounds and exercising three hours a day. I learned that I could not out train a poor diet.

And to complicate matters, my poor self-image was affecting my outlook on life and was soon causing problems in my relationships with friends and family and in my career.

When I reached out to another personal trainer to help me lose the weight and achieve the physique I had always wanted, the price was over five times the amount I had initially paid. One thing was evident—my poor food choices were now costly.

I needed a life "makeover."

I decided to forgo working with the trainer because I had been down that path. I realized that changing my lifestyle would have to start with me.

I went to a half-price bookstore and nearly purchased and read every book about nutrition. With my newfound knowledge, I did four important things:

ONE

Set a physique goal, not a weight goal. The mirror would be judge and jury, not a scale. By not focusing on what a scale told me, I freed myself from the compulsion to "hop on" several times a day to see if I was making progress. The way my clothes fit, how much energy I had, how much weight I could lift, and the way I felt about myself would better determine my progress. When I let go of the scale, I let go of a lot of my anxiety.

TWO

Started experimenting in the kitchen. I turned my kitchen into my personal "home gym." I wore my headphones to simulate a workout environment. My groceries became "the weights" and the oven and stove were the "machines." Then I started tossing food in a skillet (while fist pumping to the music) and experimenting with food combinations, with minimal seasonings, in order to teach myself what real food tasted like and so that I could learn how to pair it with other items.

> To get started, I would take some of my favorite hi-calorie meals—*such as beef fajitas, fried chicken, fried plantains, burgers, and fries*—reduce them to their core ingredients, and then find viable, healthier, and affordable alternatives for each of those ingredients.

THREE

Spent a few moments each day working on my personal development and mental health through devotionals. During that time in my life, I felt the world was "ganging up on me." I was argumentative, combative, and pretty defensive. When I stopped for a moment to reflect, I realized that the problem really wasn't everyone else. It was me. How I felt about myself was influencing my interactions, and if I wanted to succeed in other areas of life, I would need to change my attitude. My mother always told my brother and me, "Your attitude determines your altitude. You can soar with eagles or scratch with the chickens."

Around the same time, my pastor, Bishop T.D. Jakes, remarked one Sunday, "Every change you make will begin in your mind." Needless to say, I took it as a sign. My physical transformation would not be complete without getting my mind and attitude in check as well, which meant dealing with some pride and stubbornness.

Understanding that, I realized there were direct links between food, fitness, and faith. And by challenging myself in each of those areas, I could live a more fulfilled and "purpose-driven" life.

> I kept three journals or logs: 1) one to track my progress in the gym, complete with my lifting stats, workouts, and new exercises; 2) one in the kitchen to track recipes I had created and enjoyed; and 3) one for introspection that I used to track my thoughts and things that I was discovering about myself.

Each day I would set aside at least 15 minutes to spend time reading a self-improvement book, a devotional, or even a blog about a topic I was interested in. Just like I was feeding and training my body, now I was feeding and training my mind, and the more I fed my mind, the more I saw myself begin to grow and mature in other aspects of life.

FOUR

Shared my journey with others (in social media). It was social media that caused me to take a critical look at myself, and now it was social media that was going to help "fuel" my journey.

> I created accounts on Tumblr and Instagram to chronicle my journey so that I could: 1) remain accountable and focused on achieving my goals; and 2) create a vibrant community around healthy eating and living.

My objective was simple—"I share, then you share." And then pretty soon, we have a collection of ideas that can help all of us take our lives to the next level and lead to lasting, sustainable change.

I'm not saying that you should create your own blog or use social media to publicly share your journey. I am saying that you should not just keep it to yourself. Sharing it with others will help keep you motivated, enthusiastic, and optimistic at the road ahead. And most importantly, it will ensure that your "learning" is never ending.

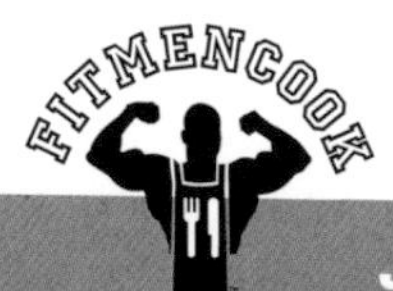

How to Use This Book

This book is meant to recreate that process for you. Whether you are where I was a few years ago, or whether you are pretty mature in your fitness and nutrition journey, something can be gained by walking through this book.

Each week is designed to help challenge you both in the kitchen and in your mind so that you transform holistically and continually.

Each day there is a devotion and accompanying recipe. The recipes are a mix of personal favorites and ones that my followers in social media have enjoyed, recreated, and shared widely with others.

Your task is simple—complete the daily devotionals and the suggested challenges each week, then fill in your Weekly Challenge Checklist, tally your score, and challenge your friends and family members to see who can get the most points.

This is not a meal-planning book. This is not a personalized diet plan. This book is designed to help you become more familiar with your kitchen and healthy cooking, while at the same time challenging you to grow both mentally and spiritually.

I invite you to take the leap countless of others around the world have already made to make healthier, wiser, and more creative decisions when it comes to food choices. If you're up for the challenge, let's get started! BOOM!

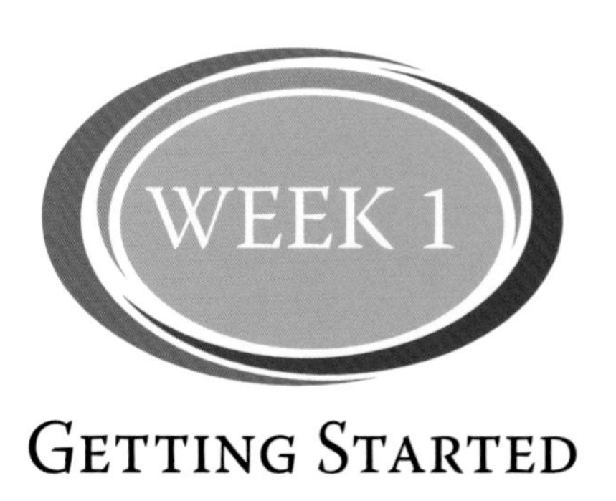

Getting Started

Challenges:

- Spend at least 10 minutes to complete the daily devotional.
- Select 2 recipes from Week 1 and prepare them.
- Find one new way to marginally increase your amount of daily physical activity for 4 of 7 days, and maintain it for the rest of the 6 weeks.
- Baseline where you are now, so you can plan where to go:
    - body fat percentage
    - strength in certain exercises
    - blood pressure
    - waist size
- Remember to adjust all recipes and portion sizes to complement your dietary needs and fitness goals.

DAY 1
Nourish Your Mind

Your
STRONGEST
MUSCLE
and your
worst enemy is your
MIND.

Train it well.

One of the things I've realized is that our life journeys, as well as our bodies, are the sum of the choices we make every day. And by and large, most of those decisions are based off the small "voice" in our head and what it whispers in our ears to either make us feel powerful, or make us feel defeated.

Because that is true, your mind is the strongest muscle and deserves adequate attention. How do you let it rest? How do you strengthen it? How do you nourish it?

Take a few moments and think about the small ways you can do this. Strengthen it by "choosing the apple over the cookie." Nourish it by "speaking well of yourself." Let it rest by regularly "removing all distractions."

And when this is done . . . Your life will be fuller. Your workouts will be grander. And you'll be ready for the next phase of your (fitness) journey.

What is your next phase?

....

....

....

....

....

....

....

....

....

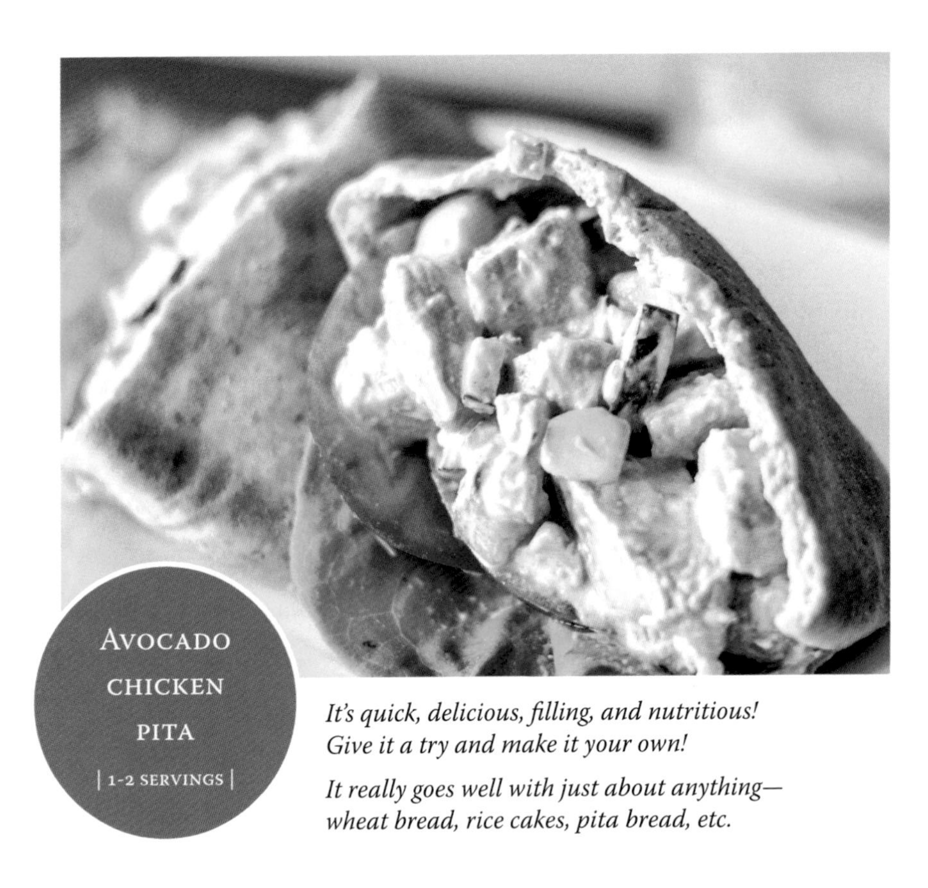

Avocado chicken pita

| 1-2 servings |

It's quick, delicious, filling, and nutritious! Give it a try and make it your own!

It really goes well with just about anything—wheat bread, rice cakes, pita bread, etc.

Ingredients

6 oz chicken breast
1 whole wheat pita
1.5 tbsp Greek yogurt
1/2 avocado
1/4 cucumber
1/4 cup red onions
tomato slices, lettuce

Seasonings

garlic, cumin, sea salt, and pepper to taste

STEPS

Season chicken breast and cook in a nonstick skillet.

Once it is finished, chop chicken into pieces.

In a bowl, mix Greek yogurt, chopped avocado, cucumber, and red onions.

Add chicken to the bowl and mix.

Add tomato slices and lettuce to the pita and stuff with the chicken salad.

Macronutrients | 452 calories, 46g protein, 38g carbs, 15g fat

DAY 2
ENTHUSIASM

The task ahead of you is never greater than the STRENGTH **within you.**

—Author Unknown

Pressure, stress, disappointment—if you have a pulse, you know the constant toll these take on your life. If you let them, they'll squeeze and drain the last drops of passion and enthusiasm out of your life. I remember feeling a bit discouraged early in my fitness journey because my body was not changing as quickly as I hoped. Whatever excitement I had about transforming my physique was shriveling up like a prune. I found myself dreading my workouts, despising my diet, and simply just making it through the day. What I was once passionate about became a chore. Ever been there?

That all changed for me when I realized that I could choose to either be powerful or defeated.

When things look down and discouraging, it's time to pull out the big guns and dig deep. Take a solid look in the mirror and tell yourself that you've got what it takes to succeed since you've made it this far. Look up. This is a lifelong journey, and you are running your own race. Be excited about the life you have been given. Believe for good things today, be enthused about your dreams coming to pass, and choose to be powerful.

What can you do to ignite the strength within?

....

....

....

....

....

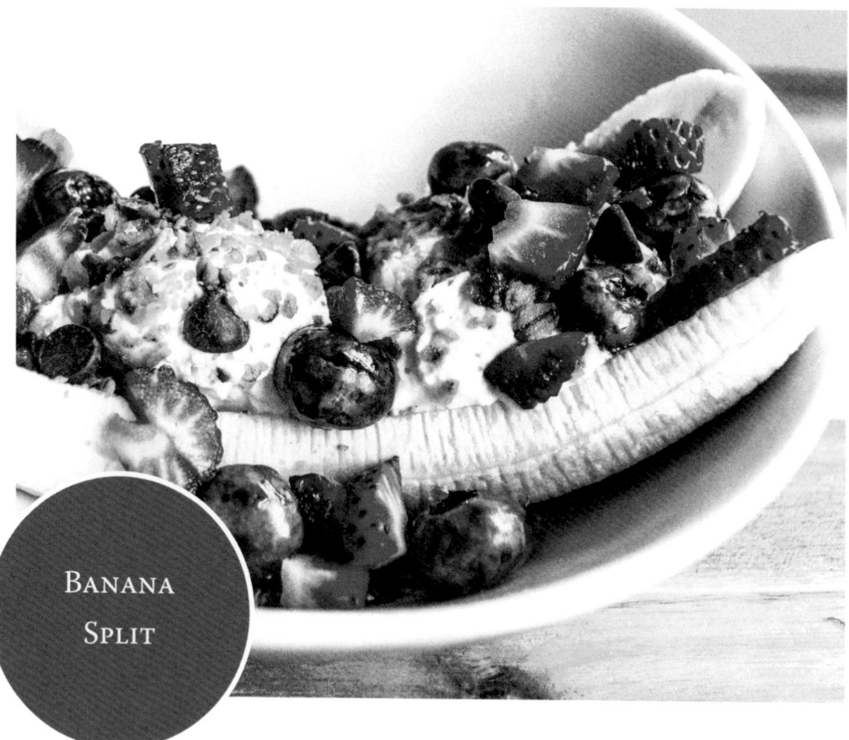

Banana Split

A great treat to enjoy first thing in the morning following a workout or brisk walk around the neighborhood.

Ingredients

1 medium banana

3/4 cup nonfat Greek yogurt

1/2 scoop vanilla isolate whey protein (no sugar, no carbohydrates)

1 strawberry

1/4 cup blueberries

1 large tbsp granola

1 tbsp dark chocolate chips

STEPS

In a bowl, mix Greek yogurt with protein powder until the texture is smooth, yet thick.

Slice a banana down the middle to divide and chop fresh fruits into small pieces.

Pour the yogurt mix on top of the banana and sprinkle the rest of the ingredients on top.

Enjoy!

Macronutrients | 383 calories, 32g protein, 53g carbs, 7g fat

DAY 3
STAY COMMITTED

A delay is not a denial.
STAY
COMMITTED.

—T.D. Jakes

One of the most frustrating things in life is waiting . . . especially on things that really matter to you, such as achieving a fitness goal, starting a new career, getting a new iPhone, finishing your degree, or maybe even finding true love. I've learned that the "easy" part is setting a goal. The "hard" part is staying committed when it appears you're not making progress.

It takes strength to get up every morning and "face the fear" that you are not where you want to be yet. And it takes faith to see that you can succeed if you don't quit.

So, no worries—just know that those six-pack abs are on the way! You want to test your true strength? Set an ambitious, realistic goal and pursue it relentlessly. This is YOUR season.

Challenge accepted? What goal will you set?

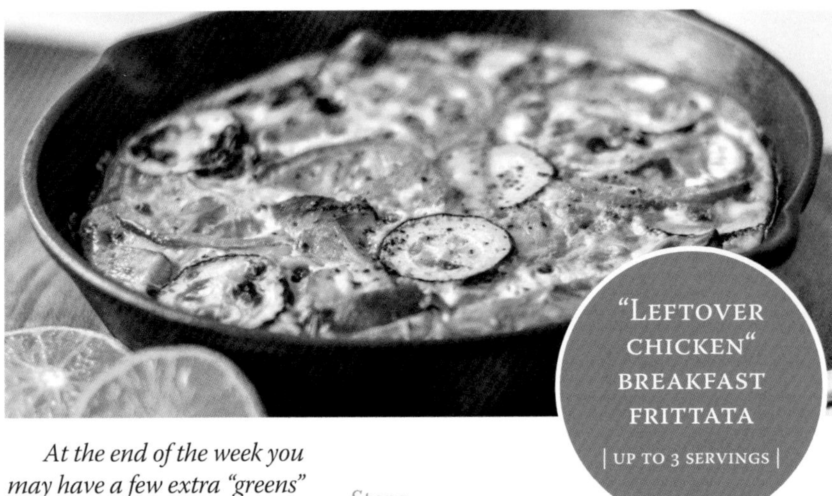

"Leftover Chicken" Breakfast Frittata

| UP TO 3 SERVINGS |

At the end of the week you may have a few extra "greens" and "proteins" that take up space in the refrigerator. Instead of tossing them away, toss them in a skillet to make a delicious and filling breakfast meal.

Ingredients

6 oz chicken breast

2 eggs

6 egg whites

250g yam

1/2 medium zucchini

1/2 Roma tomato

1/4 cup red onions

1/2 tbsp garlic paste (or minced garlic)

1 tbsp coconut oil

3/4 cup crumbled goat cheese (optional)

Seasonings

1 tsp cumin, sea salt, and pepper

Steps

Preheat the oven to 375°F.

Clean the yam by rinsing and rubbing under water, then cut it into small cubes (with skin) to allow for faster cooking.

Cut tomato into 1/3-inch pieces, then pat the slices with a paper towel to remove excess water. Chop red onion and zucchini into small pieces.

Cut the pregrilled (leftover) chicken breast into small, chunky pieces.

Add coconut oil to a cast-iron skillet and set on medium-high heat.

Once the skillet is hot, add the yam, garlic, and red onion and sear for about 5 minutes, then place the entire skillet in the preheated oven for about 15 minutes. The yam should be soft but firm.

Whisk eggs and egg whites together in a bowl. Season with cumin and paprika.

Remove the skillet from the oven and add chicken and zucchini pieces.

Pour the egg mixture over the ingredients in the skillet and top with tomato slices and goat cheese crumble if desired.

Return the skillet to the oven and bake for another 25 minutes or until the eggs have fully cooked. *BOOM!*

Macronutrients for 1 of 3 servings | 324 calories, 28g protein, 25g carbs, 4g fat

DAY 4
Small Beginnings

START

where you are.

Use what you have.

Do what you can.

—Arthur Ashe

There's a wise saying that I like to repeat to myself: Don't despise the days of small beginnings. I've had my share. The truth is that small beginnings are usually all I could handle at the time. As a child, I remember begging my parents to buy a dog. They said I was not ready, so they bought me a hamster instead. I took pretty good care of it for two weeks. Then I started to forget to feed him, clean his cage, and then the next thing you know, well . . . he passed away. Looking back, I understand the importance of starting small.

When I've started to do what I can do with what I have, I've seen some amazing things happen in my life. For two years I took photos of my food using only my iPhone, and I only upgraded to a camera so that I could make videos.

Be faithful with what you have, even when it seems small and insignificant. You never know the seeds you are planting in your life, or the life of others.

What can you do to start right where you are?

....

....

....

....

....

....

....

....

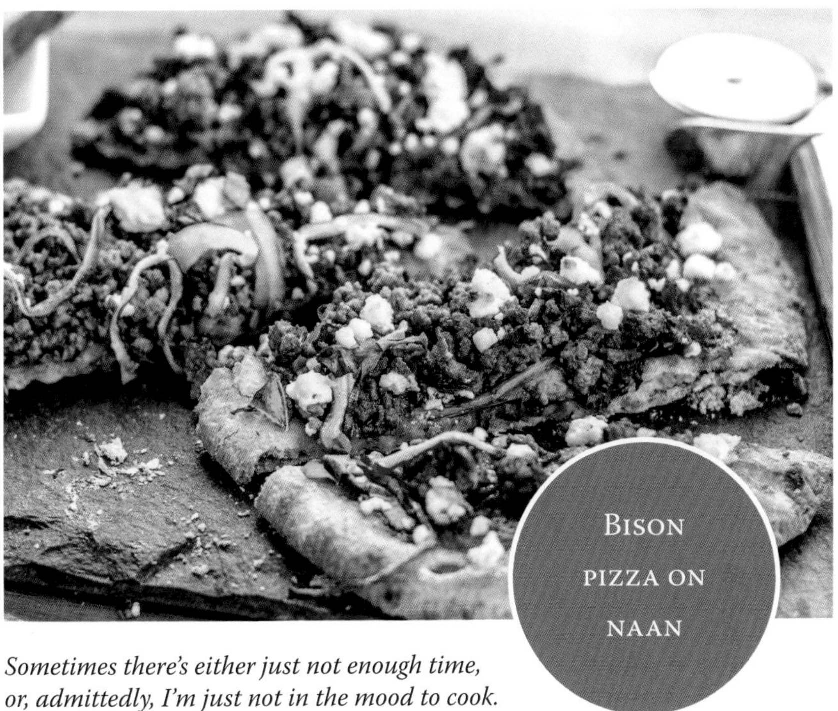

Bison pizza on naan

Sometimes there's either just not enough time, or, admittedly, I'm just not in the mood to cook. We've all experienced those moments. So one product I always keep in my freezer is whole wheat naan bread. Not only is it delicious, but it's also a healthy complex carbohydrate that I can use to make a faux-pizza. Great time-saver, no hassle, and family-approved.

Ingredients

- 1 piece wheat naan
- 6 oz lean ground bison
- 1/4 cup red onion
- 1 cup chopped spinach
- 2 tbsp Annie's Naturals Organic BBQ Sauce
- 1 oz goat cheese

STEPS

Preheat oven to 395°F.

Season and cook ground bison in a skillet with cayenne pepper, paprika, cumin, and pepper.

Spread BBQ sauce on naan bread, then add spinach.

Place cooked ground bison on a piece of naan bread.

Top with chopped or thinly sliced red onions and goat cheese.

Place the naan bread on a baking rack (so that the bottom does not get soggy).

Bake in the oven for about 20 minutes.

Macronutrients | 528 calories, 48g protein, 45g carbs, 18g fat (only 5g from bison)

DAY 5
Make a Change

You'll never
CHANGE
what you tolerate.
—Joel Osteen

I was in line at Starbucks recently. In front of me were a mother and her son. He wanted some cake, but she said no, because he apparently already had had some sweets. The little boy proceeded to throw a tantrum worthy of an Oscar. He screamed and whined until his mother finally caved in. *(And truthfully, all of us in line were just happy that a decision had been made since it was keeping us from ordering.)*

My first thought was that the kid was lucky because had I pulled this stunt as a child, my parents would've promptly beat my . . . well, you know. But it was obvious that, for whatever reason, the mom was not tired enough of his behavior to deal with it.

Then I asked myself, "What behavior or habit am I tolerating that is not helping me move forward?"

You'll never be able to lose the weight, win the race, start the company, or have peace in a relationship by tolerating mediocrity. Be tired enough to make a change. Otherwise, you'll wake up ten years later with a bratty, spoiled, and fully matured problem . . . and no progress.

What are you tolerating in your life that needs to change?

....

....

....

....

....

....

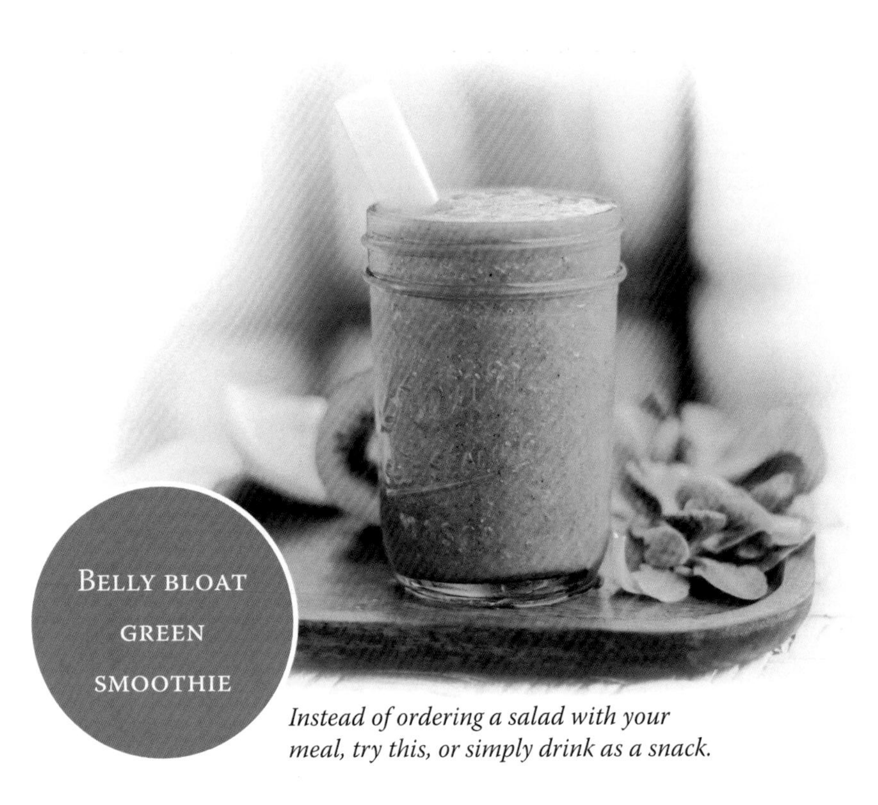

Belly bloat green smoothie

Instead of ordering a salad with your meal, try this, or simply drink as a snack.

Ingredients

1 cup spinach

1/4 cucumber

1/2 cup green tea or water

1 celery stalk

1 kiwi (optional: use 1/2 green apple and 1 slice of pineapple instead of kiwi)

Juice of 1 lemon

STEPS

Add ingredients to a blender.

Simply pulse blend for about 1 minute to ensure you remove any chunks, then blend until smooth.

BENEFITS

- Helps with digestion
- Ensures you're getting a daily serving of raw vegetables
- Helps reduce bloating
- Increases metabolism and fat-burning process

Macronutrients | 66 calories, 2g protein, 15g carbs, 0g fat

DAY 6
Stop Looking Back

Sometimes people
with the worst pasts
end up creating the
BEST
FUTURES.

—Author Unknown

It's scary to know that we can allow our past failures to leave us feeling utterly hopeless about our future. I hear someone say, "I'll feel guilty about that for the rest of my life" or "I'll never get over what I've done." Then I hear another person wallowing in their past, blaming where they are today on setbacks and heartaches that happened long ago.

Here's some good news for your future: Today is a brand-new day. Don't let your past keep you from creating a marvelous future. Stop focusing on what you can't do a thing about today. If there are things in your past that make you feel guilty, confront and deal with them. This is especially important when it comes to building a healthy lifestyle and diet. There will be moments when you may not make the best choice when it comes to your health. Recognize what happened, shrug it off, and then move on. Trust when I say this that there is so much goodness and potential inside of you—it'd be a shame if you let a little guilt stop you from sharing it with the world.

What issues from your past do you need to confront?

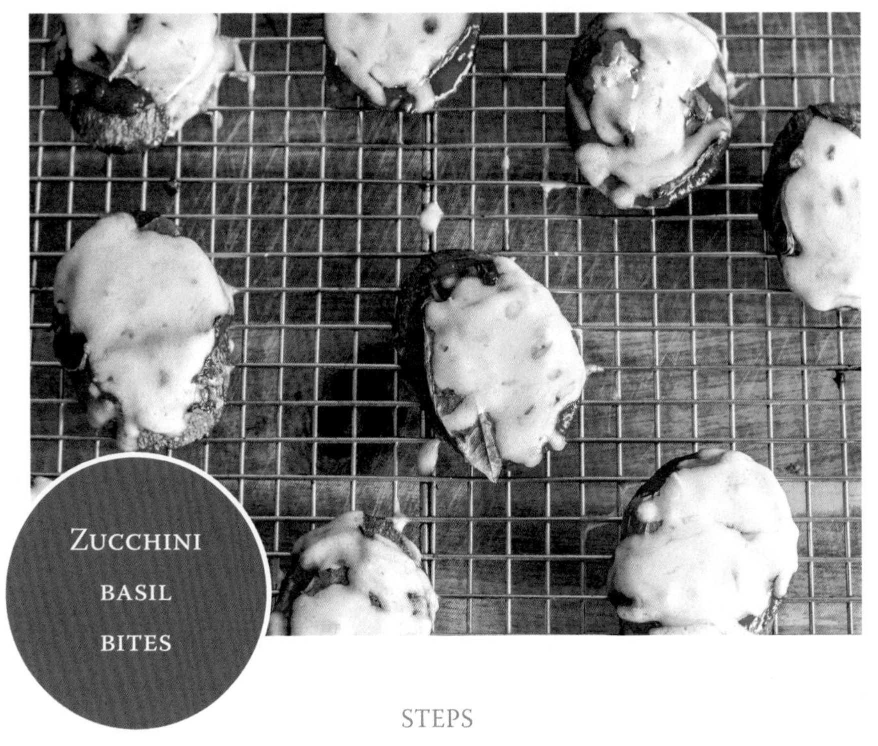

Zucchini basil bites

Ingredients

1 zucchini

2/3 cup low sodium marinara

1/3 cup mozzarella

fresh basil

1 tbsp garlic paste (optional)

STEPS

Slice zucchini into thick pieces.

Set skillet to medium-high heat.

Spray skillet with coconut oil.

Add 1 tbsp of garlic paste to skillet.

Sauté zucchini pieces for 1 minute on each side.

Remove zucchini pieces from skillet and place on a baking sheet.

On each zucchini piece add 1 tsp of marinara, then a basil leaf, then a tsp of mozzarella.

Bake for 6 minutes at 375°F.

Macronutrients per batch | 165 calories, 11g protein, 16g carbs, 7g fat

DAY 7
Do It Afraid

When you feed fear,

you starve your

FAITH.

—T.D. Jakes

A while ago my cousin asked me a question that I often think about but never really voice. He asked, "Do you ever get scared?" Without even thinking, I said, "Absolutely!" There are several things that scare me in life.

But I learned a long time ago that sometimes you have to "do it afraid," a phrase that has stuck with me after I heard a motivational speaker say it.

You can be afraid but do it anyway . . . whether it involves finishing a fitness goal that you quit too early, or changing careers because you are scared to fail, or even pursuing a relationship because you fear rejection. Whatever makes you fearful, you need to feed your faith so you can have strength to overcome. And here's the key—you can only "feed faith" by trying.

How will you feed your faith?

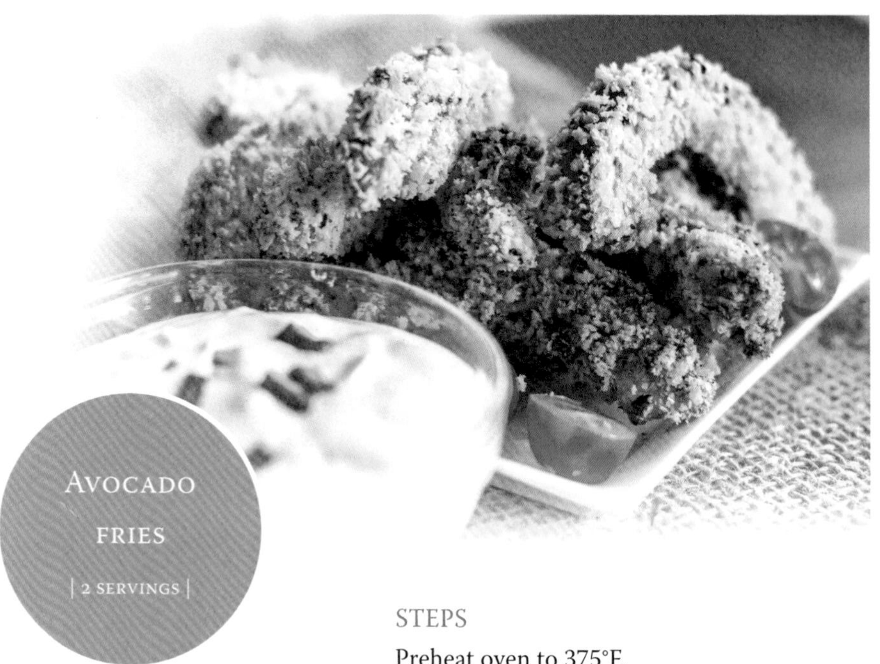

Avocado fries

| 2 servings |

Ingredients for the avocado fries

1 medium-sized avocado (medium ripe, not fully ripe)

1/2 cup panko crumbs or homemade bread crumbs

1 egg white

1 tsp Mrs. Dash seasoning, your choice of flavor

For the dipping sauce

1 tsp chopped garlic

1/2 cup Greek yogurt

1–2 tbsp lime juice

2 tsp chopped cilantro (optional)

Sea salt and pepper to taste

STEPS

Preheat oven to 375°F.

Remove the pit from the avocado.

Slice the avocado in even wedge shape slices (about 5 per half avocado) and remove the skin, if necessary with the help of a spoon.

In a bowl, mix panko crumbs and Mrs. Dash seasonings. In another bowl, whisk the egg white.

Dip the avocado slices in the egg white, then in the seasoned panko crumbs, and place them on a baking tray. Spray the slices with coconut oil spray for extra crispiness when baking.

Bake in the preheated oven for 25 minutes. Check the fries halfway and flip the wedges to get an even, golden brown and crispy coating.

To prepare the dip, mix all ingredients in a bowl and season with sea salt and pepper.

Serve the avocado fries with the yogurt dip.

Note: panko crumbs give a nice crispy coating, so try to use those if you can. If you are unable to find panko crumbs, substitute with homemade bread crumbs made from wheat bread.

Approx. macronutrients per serving (1/2 avocado) | 185 calories, 4g protein, 14g carbs, 12g fat

WEEK 1 WRAP

1. What recipes did you try this week?

2. What did you like about the recipes?

3. What would you change next time?

4. What new food item did you incorporate in your diet this week?

5. What new way did you increase your daily physical activity?

» Weekly Challenge Checklist

Completed daily devotionals?	
Prepared 2 recipes from Week 1?	
Increased daily physical activity?	
Did you baseline your health stats?	
Extra recipes created?	
Total challenges completed	

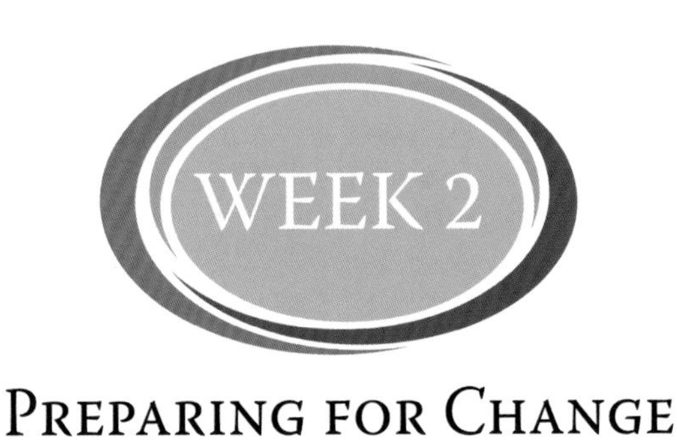

Preparing for Change

Challenges:

- Spend at least 10 minutes to complete the daily devotional.
- Select 3 recipes from Week 1 and Week 2 and prepare them.
- Select one new vegetable from the grocery store, research a healthy recipe incorporating the vegetable using FitMenCook.com or the Internet, and prepare it.
- Set a new fitness goal *(i.e. enter a race, walk/jog each day, join a kickboxing class, etc.).*
- Remember to adjust all recipes and portion sizes to complement your dietary needs and fitness goals.

DAY 1
Be Positive

You can't always PREVENT *negativity,* but you can *choose to* REMOVE IT.

One of the best things you can do for yourself is surround yourself with positive people who support you and embrace your goals. Negativity is inevitable. There will always be a different opinion or idea that could be good for you to hear. But when opinions become negative, they can be a distraction from your goals if you listen to them.

So simply remove the negative thought! Boom.

Don't waste energy trying to convince people of your intentions. If you're going to burn calories, burn them in your workout; don't waste them arguing or worrying about the negativity that may come your way.

You can start by removing that negative little voice in your head that whispers, "You can't do it." When you remove that voice, I guarantee everything else will fall into place.

What voice do you need to silence?

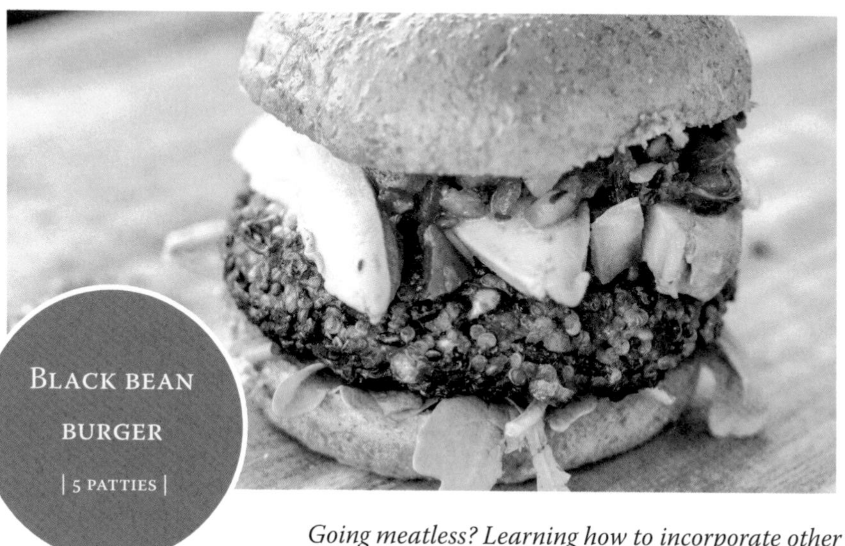

Black bean burger

| 5 patties |

Going meatless? Learning how to incorporate other nutrient-dense foods, beyond the usual ground chicken or beef or grilled salmon, is a viable way to ensure your diet remains fresh. Like these black bean and quinoa burgers! They are packed with protein, carbs, veggies, and spices to not only make you fall in love with burgers again, but also to help you feed that hard-earned muscle.

Ingredients

15 oz can black beans

1 cup cooked quinoa

1/3 cup cooked corn

2 green onions

1/4 cup bell pepper

1 egg

1/3 cup wheat germ (or instant oatmeal if you have an allergy)

Lettuce or spinach

1/2 small avocado

1/4 cup pico de gallo

Seasonings

1 tbsp smoked paprika, 1/2 tbsp cayenne, salt and pepper to taste

STEPS

Mash black beans in a bowl using a mallet or place them in a food processor.

In a large bowl, add in your ingredients and seasonings. Mix very well.

Form patties using your hands. If the patties are too loose, then add extra wheat germ.

If you are using an outside BBQ grill, then lightly spray the grill with coconut oil.

If you are cooking in a skillet, lightly spray a nonstick skillet with coconut oil.

Cook the burgers for 15 minutes, no need to flip them.

Top burgers with spinach/lettuce, sliced avocado, and pico de gallo.

Enjoy with whole wheat hamburger buns or lettuce wraps for a lower carb option.

Macronutrients per pattie | 164 calories, 11g protein, 28g carbs, 3g fat

DAY 2
Go Through

The best way out

is always

THROUGH.

—*Robert Frost*

For one person, it's insecurity that keeps them all bottled up inside. For another person, it's always trying to win other people's approval, and then being devastated when that doesn't happen. For other people I know, someone has hurt them deeply in the past, and the resentment and bitterness are killing them, yet forgiveness seems beyond them.

I've found that the only way out of whatever it is that has me trapped and locked up inside is to face it, go through it, and to do it powered by the truth. The truth, we're told, will set us free. I've found that when I've gone through the pain of facing the truth and change, it brought me freedom and healing and helped me move on to a new level.

What is it that you need to face and go through?

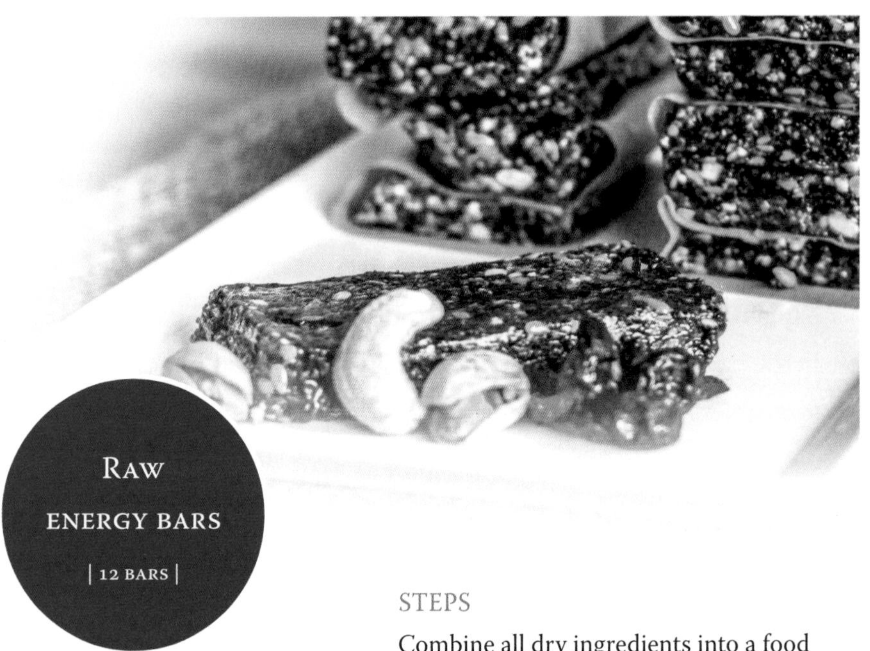

RAW ENERGY BARS

| 12 BARS |

Approximate prep and cook time: 15 minutes

Dry ingredients

1/2 cup raw pistachios

1/2 cup cashews

4 tbsp flax seeds

1/2 cup naturally dried blueberries (no sugar added)

1/2 cup naturally dried cranberries (no sugar added)

1.5 tbsp raw organic honey

1.5 tbsp (21g) coconut oil

STEPS

Combine all dry ingredients into a food processor and pulse blend until the nuts are nearly like powder, but there should be no visible pieces of nuts.

Add the remaining ingredients (dried berries, coconut oil, honey) and pulse blend until everything begins to stick together.

Pour the mixture into a bowl using a spatula and continue mixing by hand until you have malleable, sticky dough.

Spread the mixture either on a nonstick baking sheet or on parchment paper. Flatten the mixture using your hands and the spatula.

Place the pan in the freezer for 45 minutes to 1 hour, then remove.

Cut immediately into equal-sized bars and separate them using parchment paper.

Store the bars in an airtight container in the refrigerator or freezer.

Macronutrients per bar | 138 calories, 3g protein, 17g carbs, 7.5g fat

DAY 3
CHARACTER

Your physique
cannot take you
as far as your
CHARACTER.

When you look in the mirror, can you say you're leading a life of which you are proud? Yes, you may have lost a ton of weight and look amazing. Perhaps what you have been able to achieve in your physique is nothing short of amazing. That's great!

But I've learned that developing and strengthening your character counts more. Why? Because your physique and looks can never take you to places where your character cannot keep you. You will end up sabotaging your success.

I'm blessed to have friends and family members to remind me of what is more important in life. To serve others. To lead a life of integrity. To honor God by using my gifts. And to find ways to laugh more.

It is easy when undergoing so much physical change to lose sight of the important things. But never lose you. YOU are all you have. And I think you're pretty amazing.

What are you doing to strengthen your character?

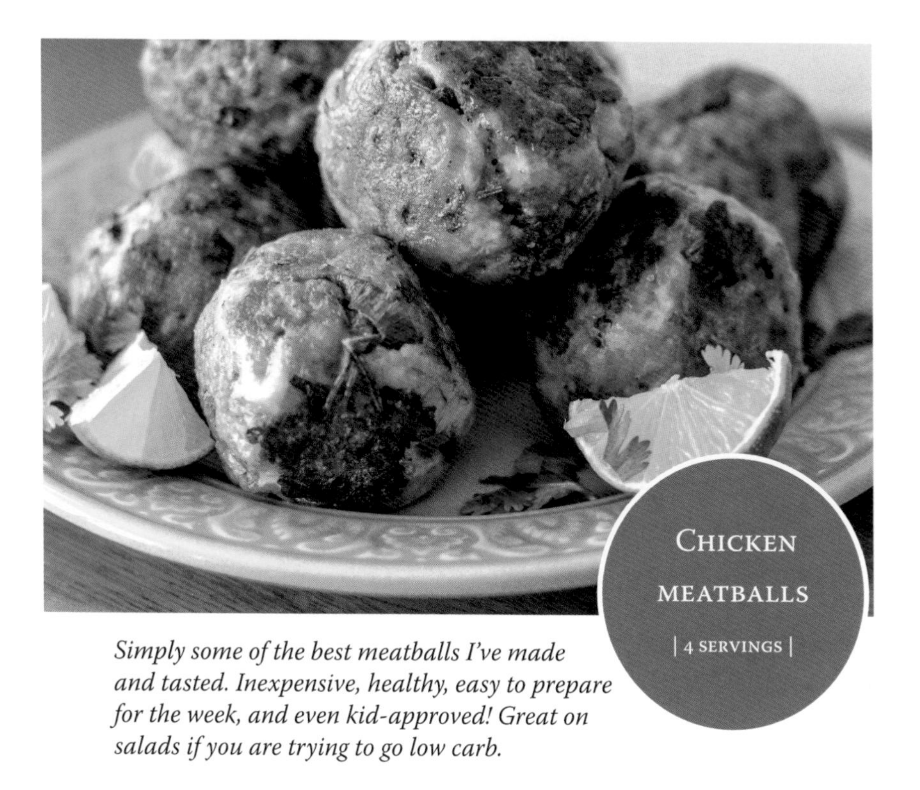

Chicken meatballs

| 4 servings |

Simply some of the best meatballs I've made and tasted. Inexpensive, healthy, easy to prepare for the week, and even kid-approved! Great on salads if you are trying to go low carb.

Ingredients

1 lb lean ground chicken (breast)

3/4 cup wheat bread crumbs

1 egg

1/3 cup chopped cilantro

1/4 cup green onions

2 fresh rosemary twigs

3/4 cup low-fat mozzarella

Seasonings

gumbo file, sea salt, pepper

STEPS

In a mixing bowl, combine all ingredients and seasonings and mix well.

Form 1–2 oz-sized meatballs.

Set a large nonstick skillet to medium-high heat.

Place meatballs in skillet and make sure to rotate them so that they are cooked through on each side.

Remove and enjoy!

Macronutrients per 1 serving | 286 calories, 34g protein, 18g carbs, 8g fat

DAY 4
Start Today

You are never too old to set another GOAL *or dream a* NEW DREAM.

—C. S. Lewis

Is there something you've wanted to do that you have been waiting to do? Perhaps you feel you've wasted so much of your life that it's too late, that you're too old to follow your dreams.

I've come to realize that if you are blessed to be able to wake up in the morning, then it is not too late to start working toward pursuing what you're passionate about. What really prompted me to start sharing my journey online was feedback from a friend. I was venting about there not being a place to find quick, healthy recipes to help people like me. She simply remarked, "So why not do it yourself?"

Don't live another day not living on purpose and following your dreams.

Be positive and look at what you have, not what you may have lost. If you have past shattered dreams, get a fresh new dream and pursue it relentlessly. *Live your dreams rather than your fears.* Make something happen today!

What dream do you need to activate today?

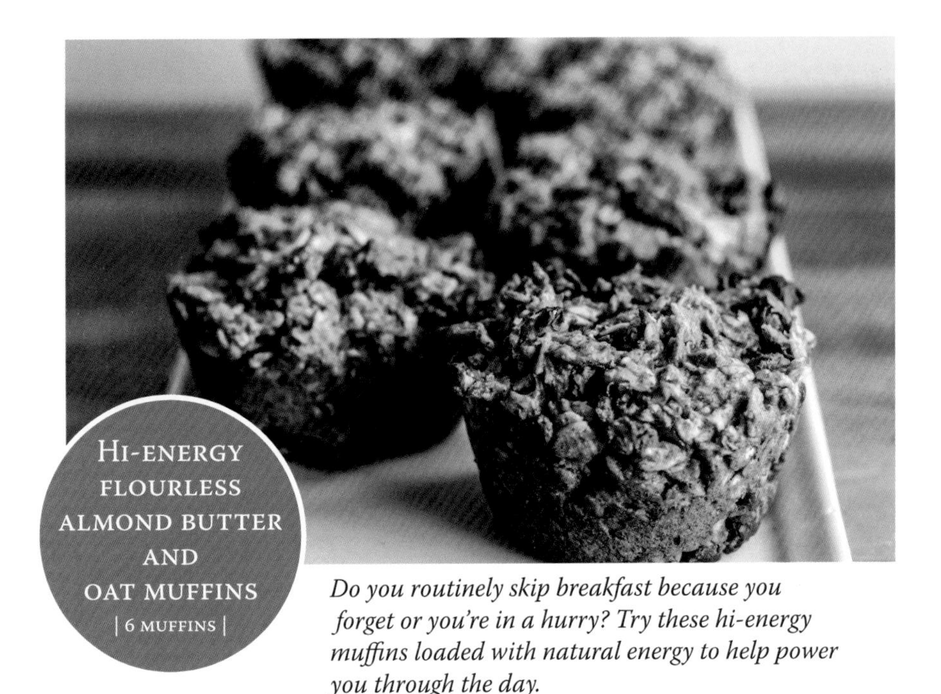

Hi-energy Flourless Almond Butter and Oat Muffins

| 6 muffins |

Do you routinely skip breakfast because you forget or you're in a hurry? Try these hi-energy muffins loaded with natural energy to help power you through the day.

Ingredients

- 2 cups rolled oats
- 1/2 cup almond butter
- 1 banana
- 4 dates
- 1/3 cup almond milk
- 1 tsp baking powder

Optional

- 1/3 cup goji berries
- 1/3 cup dark chocolate

(macronutient information does not include addition of optional ingredients)

STEPS

Set oven to 350°F.

Mix banana, dates, almond milk, and almond butter in a blender or food processor and pulse blend.

In a separate bowl, mix rolled oats and baking powder.

Add batter to the oats and mix with a rubber spatula.

Spray the muffin pan with nonstick cooking spray.

Scoop out the mixture evenly among the muffin cups.

Bake for 15 minutes at 350°F.

Macronutrients per muffin | 272 calories, 8g protein, 34g carbs, 11g fat, 6g fiber, 14g sugar

DAY 5
Understanding Strength in Silence

Silence is not abandonment.

It is a test of

STRENGTH.

The person who really got me into weightlifting was a 55-year-old man who saw me lifting weights by myself in the gym. We had nothing in common really except for our love of weightlifting. He's a great motivator, always pushing and coaching me during the workout. He's "that guy" you hear in the gym screaming at people to "push!" Initially I was a bit skeptical at his intense, focused training methods, but after seeing results, I knew there was something to be learned.

I got the chance to work out with him recently, and while he was surprised at my gains, it was business as usual. I started lifting the weights, and he did something odd. He was silent. No yelling, nothing. After each exercise, we'd just quietly move on to the next one.

I finally asked, "Hey, what's up? You're not pushing me or critiquing my form." He smiled and said, "That's 'cuz you know what you're doing." It felt incredible to hear and receive his approval.

Silence is an opportunity to show something you have learned and to test and stretch your faith. Think about it—in school, teachers are always silent during tests, and the fact that you are being tested proves you have learned something significant.

What has silence taught you?

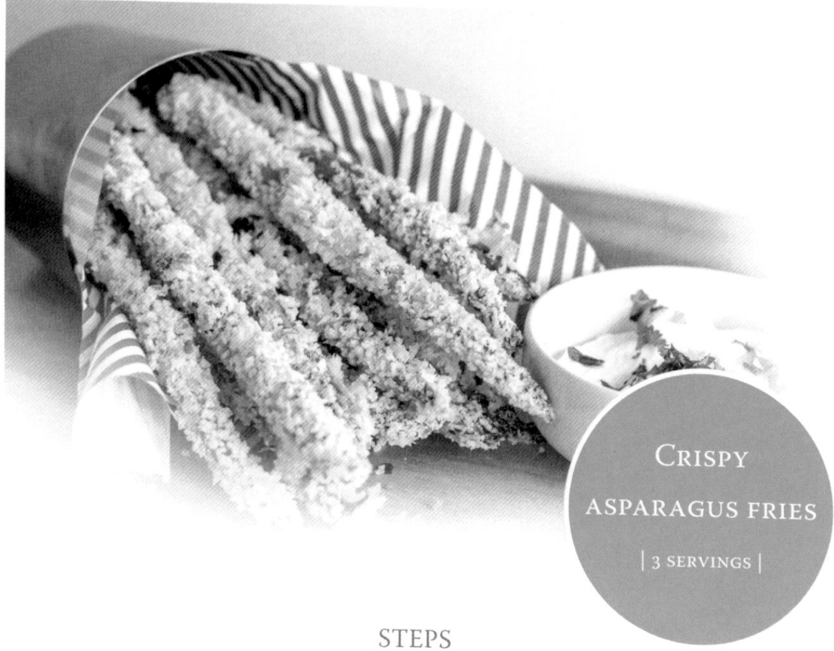

Crispy asparagus fries

| 3 servings |

Ingredients

bundle thick asparagus spears (~400g)

1 egg

1 egg white

3/4 cup panko bread crumbs

1/3 cup grated parmesan

1/4 cup coconut flour

Note: panko crumbs give a nice crispy coating, so try to use those if you can. If you are unable to find panko crumbs, substitute with homemade bread crumbs made from wheat bread.

STEPS

Preheat oven to 375°F.

In a bowl, mix panko crumbs, grated parmesan, and coconut flour. If desired, you can also add your choice of seasonings. Be careful not to add too much salt. I recommend adding sea salt once the fries are finished so you can season to taste.

In a separate bowl, whisk eggs together.

Chop the bottom stems off the asparagus and discard.

Dip the asparagus spear in the egg, then in the bread crumbs mixture.

Place the asparagus on a baking sheet lined with nonstick aluminum foil. Spray with coconut oil so the fries will be crispier upon baking.

Bake for 10 minutes at 375°F.

Approximate macronutrients per serving | 237 calories, 16g protein, 16g carbs, 9g fat

DAY 6
BE BOLD

Most obstacles
melt away
when we make up
our minds to
WALK BOLDLY
through them.

—*Orison S. Marden*

So you have some obstacles in your path. What's new? Things are not going well with your overbearing boss. Perhaps you've received some unwelcomed news from the doctor. A good friend has stopped talking to you and won't tell you why. And on top of it all, you feel like all you're doing is running in place in your life. Rather than moving forward and expecting good things ahead of you, you've allowed the obstacle to put your life on hold.

Whatever is going on in our lives, whether it's a disappointment or a setback or financial issue, I've discovered that the obstacles that stand between me and my future are what cause me to grow. I usually don't enjoy my faith and perseverance being stretched, but if I can keep the right attitude, the difficulties actually work for my good and advantage. When I have the boldness to walk through them, the barriers of my past get broken and my next level of opportunity opens.

That obstacle in your way—what will you do to walk through it?

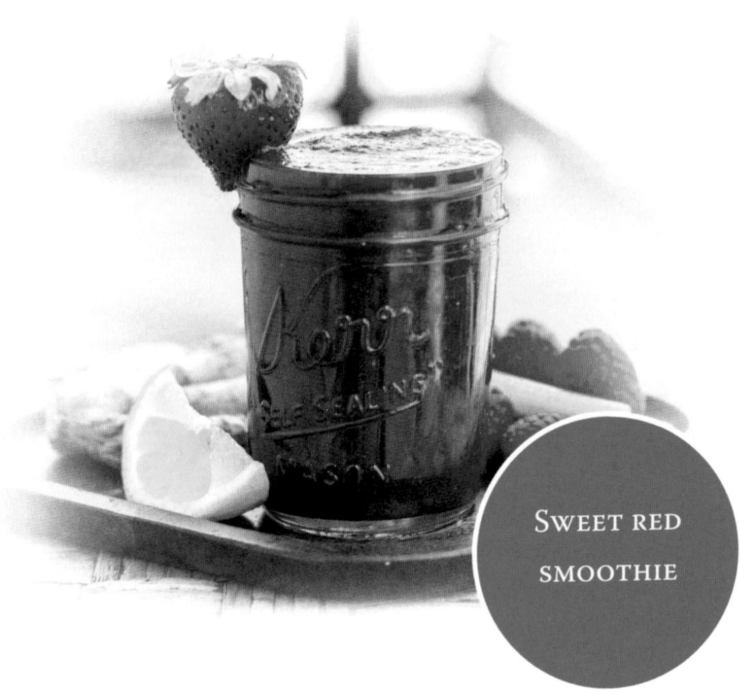

Sweet red smoothie

Ingredients	STEPS
1/2 red beet	Add ingredients listed above to a blender.
1 small red apple	Simply pulse blend for about 1 minute to ensure you remove any chunks, then blend until smooth.
1 celery stick	
3 large strawberries	Instead of ordering a salad with your meal, try this, or simply drink as a snack.
1/4 banana	
green tea (optional)	
1/3 cup raspberries (optional)	
1 tsp ginger (optional)	
Ice or water, as needed	

BENEFITS

- Beets are great for exercise as they help to improve blood flow, thereby increasing your muscular endurance
- Rich in antioxidants that aid in detoxification
- Beets help to purify the blood, reduce inflammation, and even cleanse the liver
- Regulation of blood sugar levels
- Curbs appetite and feelings of hunger

Macronutrients with the optional ingredients | 168 calories, 1g protein, 35g carbs, 1g fat

DAY 7
ABUNDANT HEALTH

The key to wholeness and wellness

is finding a

BALANCED LIFE.

Ever drive a car with unbalanced tires? It's a bumpy ride, but even worse the car tends to veer to the sides, and, over time, the tires wear unevenly and are more prone to blowouts.

The same is true for us. Many of us struggle in maintaining a balance between work and play and between obligations to others and obligations to self. Some things require effort and exertion, and other things require rest and recreation. Our challenge is to find *balance.*

The healthier you are and the more balanced your life, the more you will have a sense of total well-being. You'll feel that the quality of your life is rising. Your work will be more creative and easier, your attitude will be more positive, and your relationships will be more relaxed and loving. When that happens, virtually *everything* in your life—both tasks and relationships—is impacted in a positive way.

Pursue a life of abundant health and don't settle for anything less.

Are you pursuing or settling?

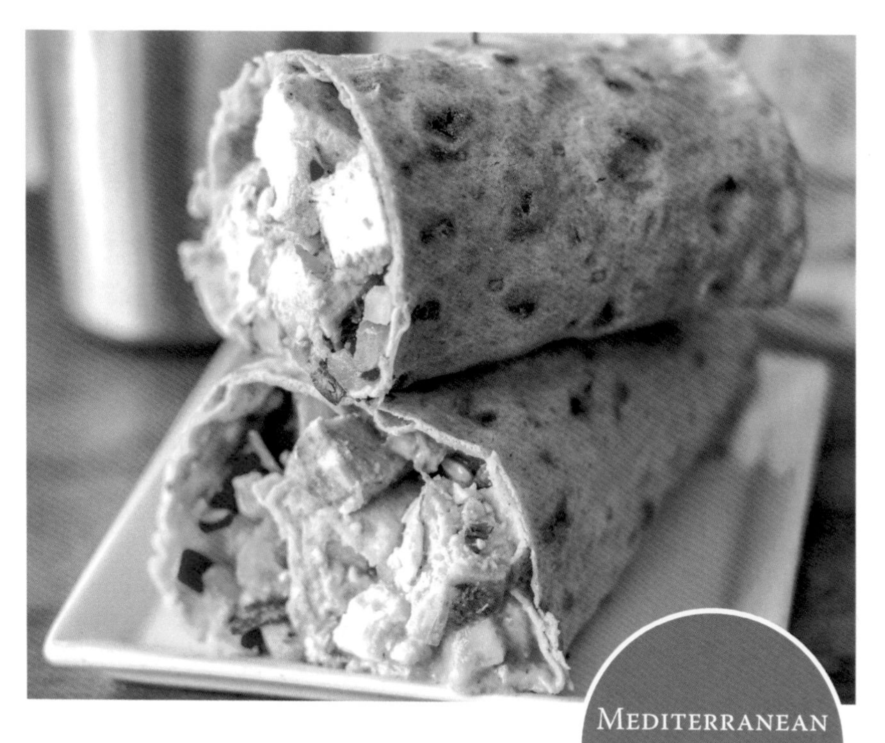

Mediterranean chicken wrap

Need a new sandwich for lunch? Try this Mediterranean-inspired chicken wrap that's easy to make, will satisfy your taste buds, and feed those muscles.

Ingredients

5 oz chicken breast

1 piece wheat lavash bread

3 tbsp hummus

1/4 cup pico de gallo

2 tbsp feta cheese

1/8 cup diced cucumber

1 celery stalk

STEPS

Set nonstick skillet to medium-high heat.

Cook chicken breast in nonstick skillet on both sides.

Cut chicken breast into cubes.

In a large mixing bowl, add chicken, pico de gallo, diced cucumber, diced celery and mix well.

Spread hummus evenly across the lavash bread.

Add the chicken mix to the lavash bread and then sprinkle the feta over the mix.

Roll up the lavash bread to make a wrap and cut it in half to make it easier to handle.

Macronutrients | 465 calories, 45g protein, 40g carbs, 12g fat

WEEK 2 WRAP

1. What recipes did you try this week?

2. What did you like about the recipes?

3. What would you change next time?

4. What new vegetable did you incorporate in your diet this week?

5. What was your new fitness goal?

» Weekly Challenge Checklist

Completed daily devotionals?	
Prepared 3 recipes from Week 1 or 2?	
Selected a new vegetable and prepared it?	
Set a new fitness goal?	
Extra recipes created?	
Total challenges completed	

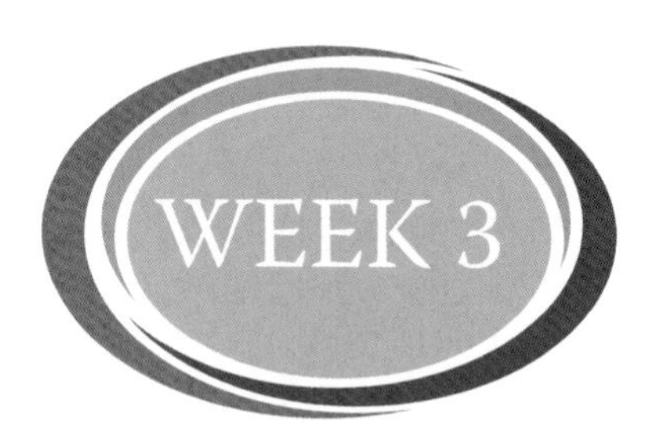

Finding Your Rhythm and Broadening Your Horizons

Challenges:

- Spend at least 10 minutes to complete the daily devotional.
- Select 4 recipes from Week 1 through Week 3 and prepare them.
- Visit and, if possible, shop at a different grocery store than the one you normally frequent.
- Select one new lean protein source (see page 157), research a healthy recipe incorporating the protein using FitMenCook.com or the Internet, and prepare it.
- Perform light stretching exercises for 15 minutes in the morning or before bed for 3 days this week, and continue for the next 3 weeks.
- Remember to adjust all recipes and portion sizes to complement your dietary needs and fitness goals.

DAY 1
FOLLOW YOUR HEART

When you stop chasing money and start CHASING PURPOSE, *you will find* PROSPERITY AND PEACE.

I recently did something radical. I quit my job. I walked away from a great-paying job with amazing benefits because of two things—passion and purpose. Oftentimes the paths we choose for ourselves do not align with our true passion and purpose. For me, those roads are safe and don't really require anything "extra" from me. But one thing I got from playing it safe was restlessness, wondering, *"What would happen if I followed my heart?"*

I spent a year juggling a full-time job and my passion for sharing healthy food. It was very difficult. I admit I was afraid to move forward because I had grown comfortable with doing what is easy.

But the day came when I decided to follow my passion by putting my all into Fit Men Cook. While I'm optimistic about the future, I do not know exactly what it holds and at times, admittedly, that can be unsettling. But I do know this: Five years from now I won't be asking myself "What if?" And knowing that helps me rest a little easier.

Where do you need to follow your heart?

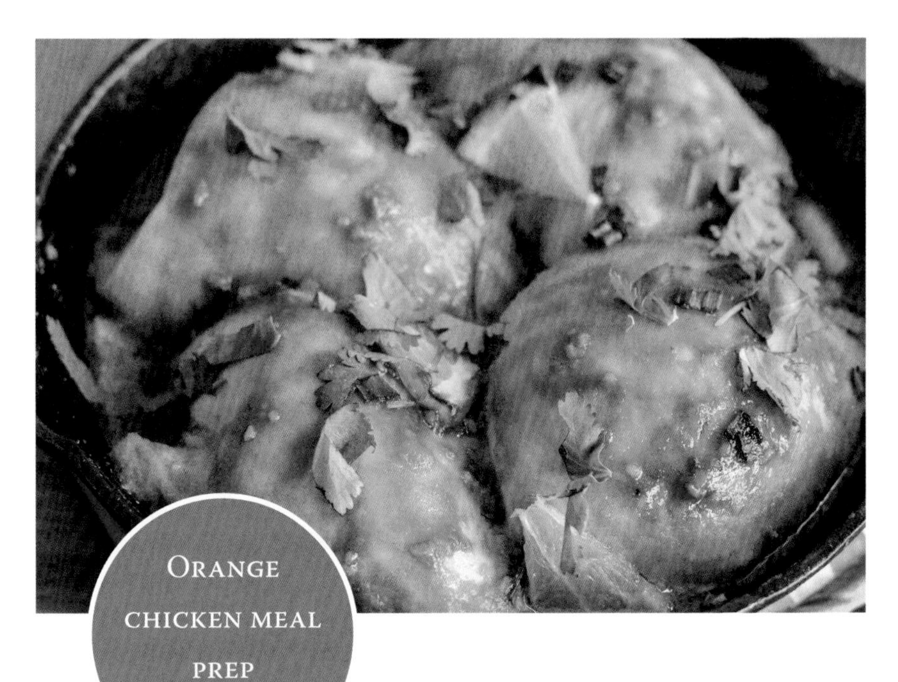

Orange chicken meal prep

| 5 servings |

Ingredients

2 lbs of chicken breast (raw)

2 tbsp hot mustard (Asian style)

2 tbsp raw honey

1 tbsp Bragg's Liquid Aminos

1 tbsp garlic

Juice from half orange

STEPS

In a large bowl, add chicken breast, mustard, garlic, honey, liquid aminos, and juice from the orange.

Mix all ingredients and let chicken marinate for at least 20–30 minutes.

Set oven to 450°F.

Place marinated chicken in heavy cast-iron skillet and bake for 20 minutes.

Remove from oven and garnish with cilantro.

Tips

Add 1 tbsp wheat or coconut flour to the sauces to thicken it (optional).

For a golden color, after baking for 20 minutes, remove chicken from the oven. Set the oven to high broil. Spoon excess sauce over the chicken and then place back in the oven and bake for 3–5 more minutes.

Macronutrients per serving | 220 calories, 42g protein, 9g carbs, 2g fat

DAY 2
Change Your Focus

If you focus on results, you will never change.

If you focus on change, you will GET RESULTS.

—Jack Dixon

When we face disappointment or disillusionment with someone or something in our lives, we realize the power that expectations have over us. We may even find this true when we think we're doing the best things. We change our thinking and start believing for something bigger and better for our lives, but then the bottom falls out. You know the feeling.

For instance, we may have had high hopes that we'd be looking trimmer after following a new eating plan for a few weeks, but the mirror shows nothing. Here's the trick: If you focus on results, even if you see initial results, it's not going to last, because you'll grow weary of it, be disappointed, and go back to your old ways. But if you'll focus on changing your lifestyle to one of eating wisely, you change your motivation and tap into the power that will eventually bring the results you are looking for, and it will last!

Disappointed? Disillusioned? Where do you need to change your focus?

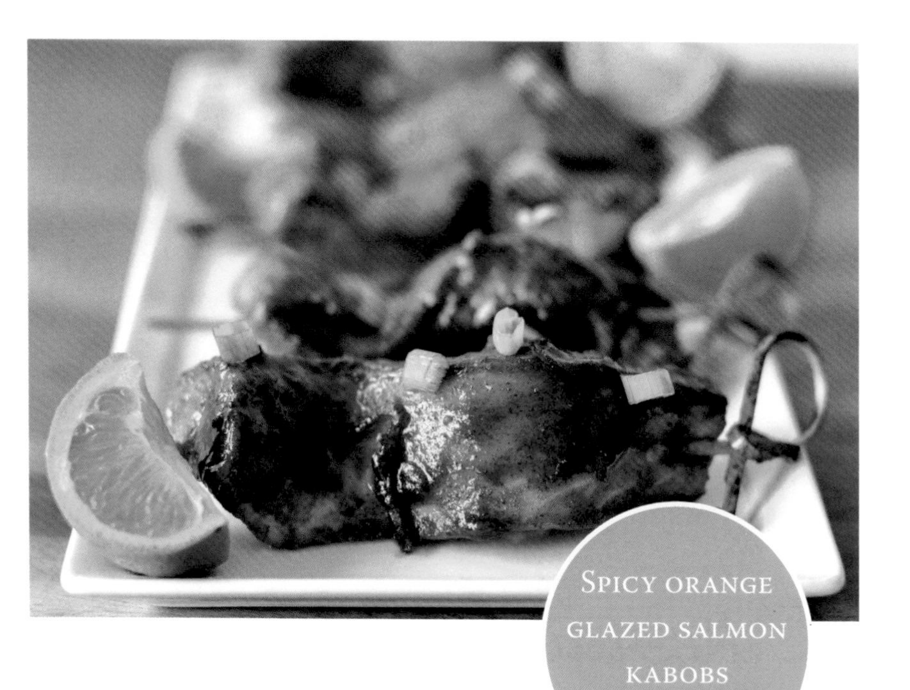

Spicy orange glazed salmon kabobs

| 3-6 servings |

Here's a quick and delicious way to freshen up your next recipe if the spices you normally use are tasting a little "stale." And the good thing about this marinade is that it is versatile and can be used on other proteins and vegetables alike.

Ingredients

1/4 cup sugar free orange marmalade

1/2 tbsp paprika

1/2 tbsp coconut sugar

1 tsp Tabasco (or 1 tsp cayenne pepper)

Juice from 1 mandarin orange

STEPS

Preheat oven to 405°F.

In a bowl, mix orange marmalade, paprika, coconut sugar, Tabasco sauce, and freshly squeezed orange juice.

Slice salmon into 2–3 oz pieces for the kabobs.

Add salmon pieces to marinade and let it marinate for 20 minutes (no more than 45 minutes).

Skewer salmon with kabob sticks.

Bake in the oven for 8–10 minutes at 405°F.

Macronutrients for ENTIRE batch | 81 calories, 0g protein, 30g carbs, 0g fat

DAY 3
Letting Go

Stop chasing people
who hurt you.

Replace them
with people

WHO CARE.

Are you using fitness to "chase someone"? I'll confess—yes, I did! Don't judge me! There's nothing like a broken heart to help you start exercising. "Can I get an Amen?" Ha!

At some point along "the chase," something strange happened. I relapsed and gained back all the weight . . . and more! And I soon realized that my broken heart was not enough to carry me through a lifetime of fitness. While the heartache got me started, it couldn't keep me going. I had to make a change for me.

So I decided to stop "chasing her" through fitness, and I allowed myself to meet other amazing people. As my heartache eventually stopped, my fitness journey kept going. And that decision to "let go" made the difference in my life.

What or who are you "chasing" that you need to let go?

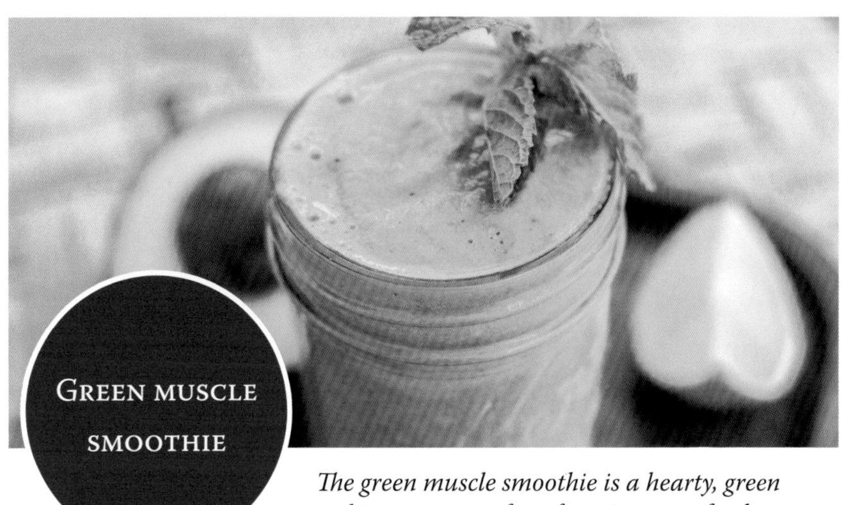

Green muscle smoothie

The green muscle smoothie is a hearty, green smoothie using two of my favorite super foods—kale and avocado. Some people avoid incorporating fats into their daily diet in hopes that they will lose weight; but, incorporating healthy fats from sources such as avocado can actually encourage fat loss since avocados have a type of sugar—mannoheptulose—that actually impedes the release of insulin.

Ingredients

2 kale leaves

1/2 small avocado

1/2 green pear

2 pineapple slices

3 strawberries

1/4 cucumber

1 mint sprig (optional)

Fresh lime juice (optional)

Ice or water, as needed

STEPS

Add ingredients listed above to a blender.

Simply pulse blend for about 1 minute to ensure you remove any chunks, then blend until smooth.

Instead of ordering a salad with your meal, try this, or simply drink as a snack.

BENEFITS

- Feeling satisfied to avoid overeating
- Boost of energy from the mono-unsaturated fats that are used by the body to slowly burn energy
- Packed with antioxidants and vitamins to support skin and cardiovascular health
- Has enzyme bromelain—found in pineapple—to serve as an anti-inflammatory to help prevent bruising, swelling, and redness
- Mint can help relieve allergy symptoms and help ease digestion

Macronutrients | 254 calories, 6g protein, 40g carbs, 12g fat

DAY 4
ENJOY YOU

I think I like
who I am becoming.
YOU

How do you feel about yourself? I haven't done a survey, but many people I meet say they don't like themselves, and for any number of reasons. Our world has created such a false, unrealistic image of what we should look like and be like. The image tends to be skinny, buffed, with a flawless complexion, perfect hair, and trendy clothes. Stay at home moms feel guilty for not having a career. Singles feel they are missing something because they are not married. Men feel worthless because their career fails to bring them great satisfaction.

I hope that you can say that you like who you are becoming. Wow! That's incredibly powerful. You may not be all you want to be, but you're not what you used to be, and you're making strides toward what you want to be. Stop looking at your faults and how far you have to go, and recall how far you've already come. You have more possibilities in you than you can even imagine. You have gifts and talents that nobody else has on this planet. You're a work in progress. Enjoy "the you" who's becoming!

How do you feel about yourself?

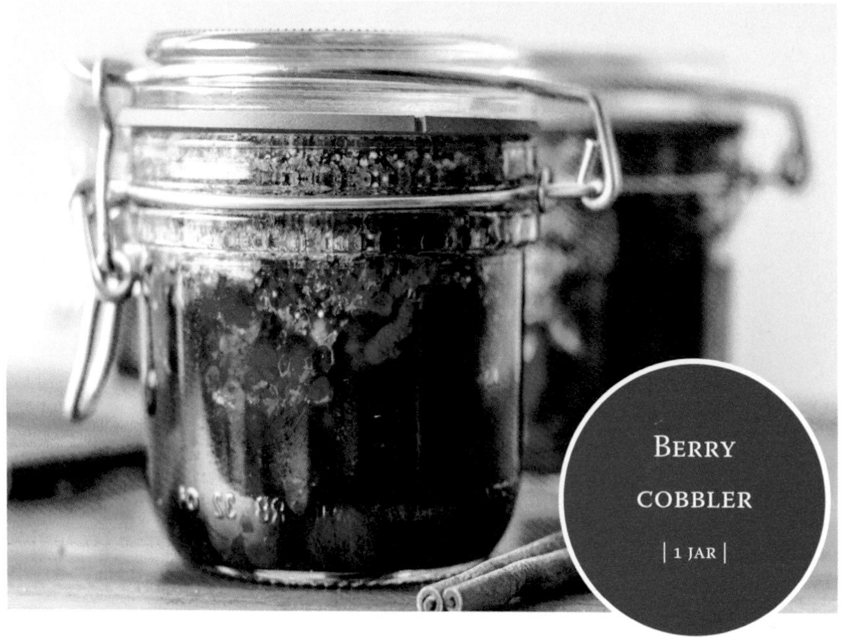

Berry cobbler

| 1 JAR |

Having meals prepared for the day and week is a proven way to help you stay on track to achieve your goals.

Ingredients

1/4 cup dry, uncooked instant oats (oatmeal)

1/4 cup blueberries

1/8 cup blackberries

1/8 cup raspberries

2 tbsp coconut flour, or 1/4 scoop vanilla isolate whey protein (no sugar, no carbohydrates)

Juice from 1/2 clementine or orange

1 tbsp cinnamon

1 tbsp coconut sugar

1 tbsp coconut oil

Utensils

7 oz hermetic jar

STEPS

Set oven to 350°F.

In a bowl, mix oats, coconut flour (or protein powder), coconut sugar, cinnamon, and melted coconut oil. Set aside.

In a small hermetic jar or mini-casserole dish, add blueberries, blackberries, and raspberries and lightly mash with a fork. Squeeze orange juice over the berries.

Top the berries with the coconut oats mixture to serve as your crust.

Repeat the process for other jars.

Spray the top of the cobbler in jars with coconut oil and bake for 25 minutes at 350°F.

Macronutrients per jar | 314 calories, 10g protein, 37g carbs, 10g fat

DAY 5
Don't Quit

FAITH.

You don't have
to see it to *believe* it.
*But you must
believe it to receive it.*

One thing I'll admit to being is stubborn when I'm told no. To me, nearly everything is negotiable. In fact, never stand behind me in line at Subway because I'm "that guy" who has a million changes to the sandwiches. I know, it's bad.

But life is not always negotiable. Sometimes you don't win. Sometimes you don't get the job. Sometimes those results in the gym are not immediately seen. And it sucks. After speaking with a friend about a recent setback, I was reminded of the importance of having faith. While circumstances may not always "appear" favorable, you must believe that things will get better. "You'll win, if you don't quit." It's hard but stay the course and walk by faith.

How do you keep yourself encouraged during difficult times?

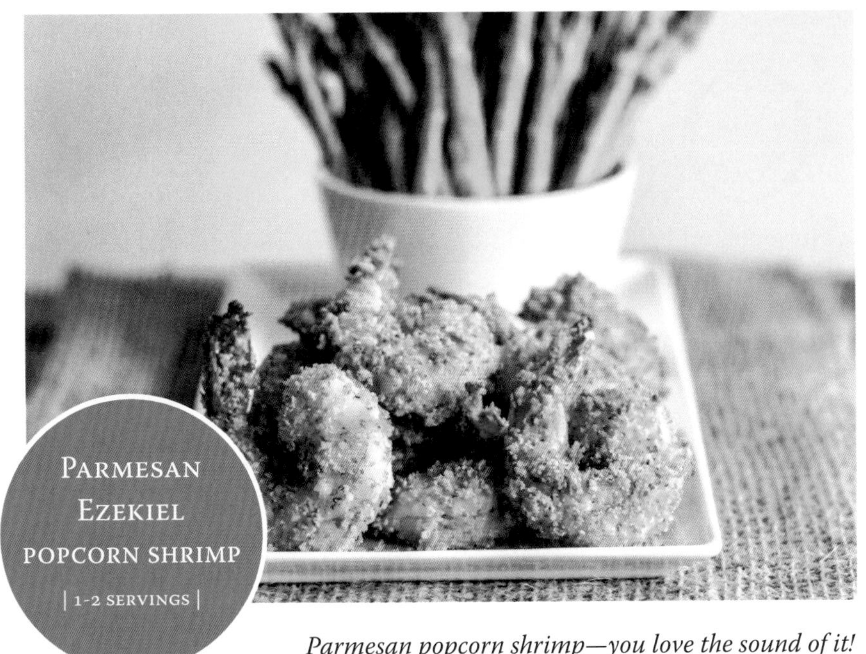

Parmesan Ezekiel popcorn shrimp

| 1-2 servings |

Parmesan popcorn shrimp—you love the sound of it! And what's more, your body will thank you for this delicious, nutritious take on a popular food that is usually covered in grease! I guarantee this is a recipe your family, especially kids, will enjoy.

Ingredients

1/2 pound raw shrimp (peeled and deveined)

2 slices whole wheat bread (or Ezekiel bread)

1/2 cup reduced fat parmesan cheese

1 egg

Seasonings for crumb batter

garlic, sea salt, Mrs. Dash, pepper

STEPS

Set oven to 375°F.

Toast pieces of bread. Add the toast to a blender or food processor to make bread crumbs.

In a bowl, mix bread crumbs, garlic, sea salt, Mrs. Dash (seasoning of your choice), pepper, and parmesan.

In another bowl, beat an egg.

Dip the raw shrimp in the egg and then into the bread crumb mixture. Place it on a baking sheet. Repeat the process until all of the pieces of shrimp are covered in bread crumbs and on the baking sheet.

Bake the shrimp in the oven for 7 minutes or until shrimp is fully cooked.

Macronutrients using Genesis bread | 520 calories, 63g protein, 34g carbs, 15g fat

DAY 6
Develop Your Strengths

STRONG

is what happens

when you

run out of weak.

—Author Unknown

If you're like me, one thing you really hate is being weak. Weak people get taken advantage of, right? So I compensated by trying to look strong and tough and independent. But the reality is that I have weaknesses and flaws, and trying to compensate for all of them just sapped the strength I did have. The day finally came when I told myself it was okay to have my weaknesses, and that I didn't have to battle them or cover them up.

I found that I had to run out of my weakness, just let them go, and concentrate on developing my strengths. While it doesn't mean I am now accepting those weaknesses as a permanent part of my life, it does mean that I no longer let the weaknesses rob my time and efforts from growing my strengths. And in doing so, I've found some of what I thought we're my big problems really were only irritations that I could finally deal with because I had become strong.

What weakness are you obsessing over that you need to let run out?

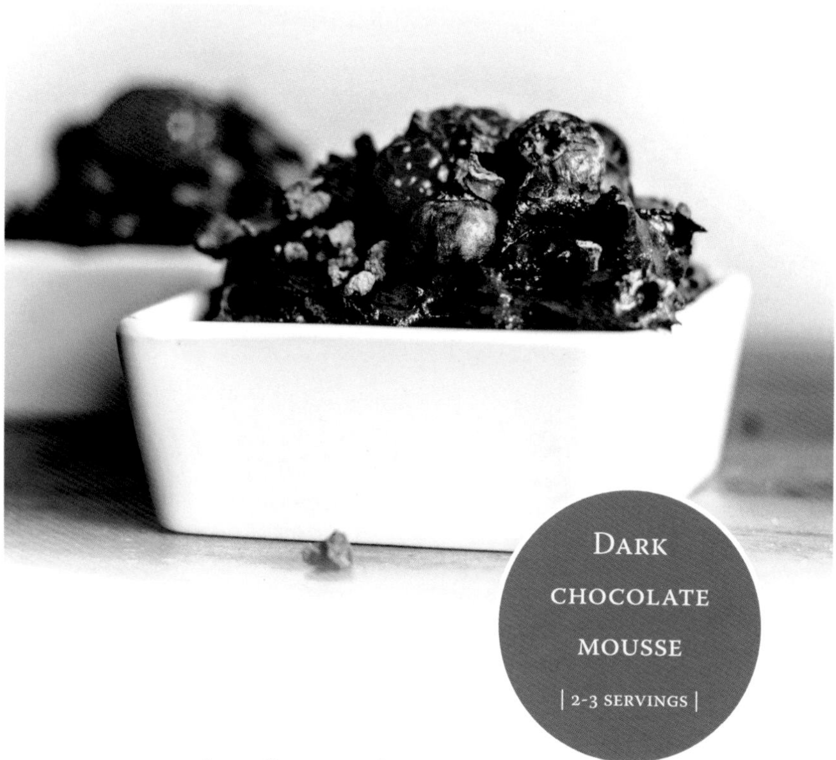

Dark chocolate mousse

| 2-3 SERVINGS |

Ingredients

2 small avocados

5 dried dates

1/4 cup cacao powder (or dark chocolate powder)

1/2 cup almond milk

STEPS

Cut avocado into halves and scoop out avocado into blender.

Add dates, cacao powder, and almond milk to blender with avocado.

Blend ingredients until consistency is smooth.

Add to serving dishes and garnish with berries and cacao nibs (optional).

Macronutrients for 3 servings | 233 calories, 4g protein, 30g carbs, 10g fat, 5g fiber

DAY 7
Sweet Success

Failure is the condiment

that gives

SUCCESS

its flavor.

—*Truman Capote*

Condiments made from natural ingredients, true delicacies that have a sweet smoothness that *delights* the palate—don't get me started on how much I love them! But I run into people all the time who are so afraid to experiment and try new flavors and add some spice to their foods. It's very much like how many of us view failure. We think that trying something and failing means we're a failure, which is absolutely false!

NBA superstar Michael Jordan was once cut from his high school basketball team. Henry Ford went broke five times before he succeeded. Fourteen book publishers rejected Max Lucado's first manuscript before one offered him a contract. Just take a failure as another door opening to where you want to go. Trial and error is the path to success, and if you refuse to give up and ultimately succeed, any failure along the way will only make the victory sweeter!

How can you change the way you deal with failure?

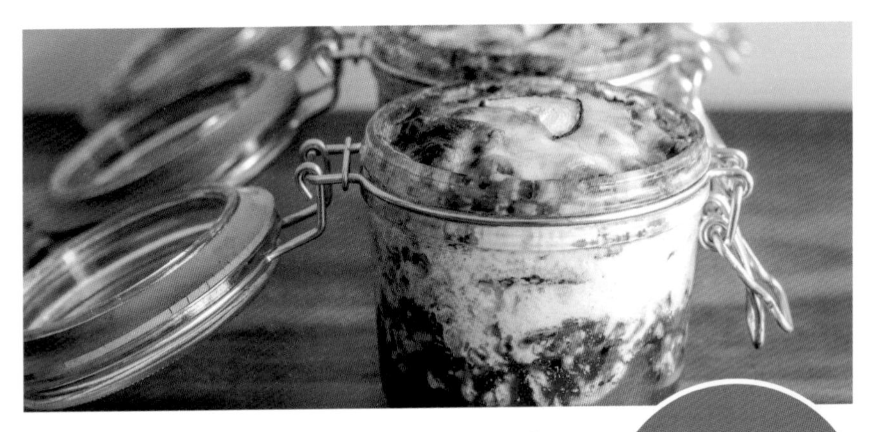

Turkey & Zuchinni Lasagna

| UP TO 6 SERVINGS |

Here's a quick spin on my hi-protein Zucchini Lasagna that will help with portion control. Raid your grandma's cabinet and grab some hermetic jars and stuff them with the lasagna ingredients. You can also find jars at your local store. This is simple, fast, and budget friendly.

Hermetic jars: simply remove the metal ring and reheat in the microwave or in the oven. And since hermetic jars are airtight, these store and freeze well so you can enjoy throughout the week.

Ingredients

1 lb extra lean ground turkey

1.5 cup low sodium basil marinara sauce (I used Trader Joe brand)

1 zucchini

1 cup low-fat cottage cheese

1 egg white

1/3 cup chopped red onion

3/4 cup reduced fat mozzarella (optional but recommended)

Seasonings for meat

garlic powder, onion powder, cumin

Seasoning may not be needed if you purchase a "seasoned" marinara sauce.

STEPS

Preheat oven to 350°F.

In a nonstick skillet set to medium-high heat, cook ground turkey with marinara sauce and chopped red onion until meat is done.

Slice zucchini into pieces using a knife or a mandolin.

In a bowl, mix cottage cheese with egg white.

In hermetic jar, add a layer of zucchini slices at the bottom, followed by the meat sauce mix, and then add cottage cheese/egg mix. Repeat this process with zucchini and meat sauce. Top it all off with a 1/4 cup of mozzarella.

Repeat above process for 2 additional jars.

Bake in the oven for 30 minutes at 350°F.

Enjoy!

Macronutrients per serving (about 5 oz turkey) | 387 calories, 55g protein, 16g carbs, 12g fat

WEEK 3 WRAP

1. What recipes did you try this week?

2. What did you like about the recipes?

3. What would you change next time?

4. What new grocery store did you visit this week?

5. What new protein source did you choose and what meal did you prepare with it?

6. How did it feel to incorporate stretching into your regimen?

» Weekly Challenge Checklist

Completed daily devotionals?	
Prepared 4 recipes from Week 1–3?	
Visit and shop at a new grocery store?	
Selected a new protein and prepared it?	
Incorporated light stretching 3x this week?	
Extra recipes created?	
Total challenges completed	

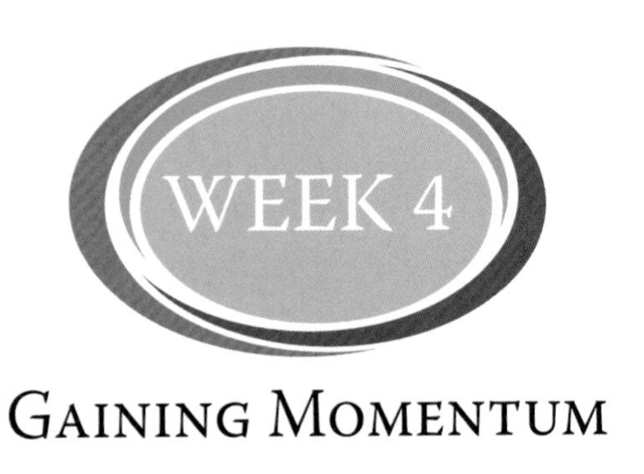

Gaining Momentum

Challenges:

- Spend at least 10 minutes to complete the daily devotional.
- Select 5 recipes from Week 1 through Week 4 and prepare them.
- Make two natural fruit and vegetable smoothies.
- Select one power food or complex carbohydrate (see page 156), research a healthy recipe incorporating the ingredient using FitMenCook.com or the Internet, and prepare it.
- Increase your water consumption or non-sugary liquids. Aim for about 10–12 cups of water per day. Very active individuals—performing more than 1 hour of strenuous athletic activity—should aim to consume more to compensate for the amount of sweat (fluid) loss during exercise and daily activities.
- Remember to adjust all recipes and portion sizes to complement your dietary needs and fitness goals.

DAY 1
Speak Positively

If you cannot be

POSITIVE,

then at least be quiet.

—Joel Osteen

I admit that I am not always positive. I've got this "hater" called "my mind," and he can be pretty annoying. Despite the positive things that happen in my life, he always seems to find something negative to say. Does your mind ever play these tricks on you?

Haters say things such as, "You don't have what it takes." Or "That fitness goal is impossible." Or "You'll never get that career."

Recently, I was reminded of something my mother taught me: "You have to speak well of yourself so that you can begin to believe it FOR yourself." At times we will doubt. But I am convinced that when you speak positively, you will begin to see hope in your situations and find strength to overcome.

So if you're worried about that weight, walk up to the mirror, hit a quick flex, and say, "Yo, you lookin' good, homie!"

And if you cannot be positive, then just be quiet until you can be.

How do you encourage yourself?

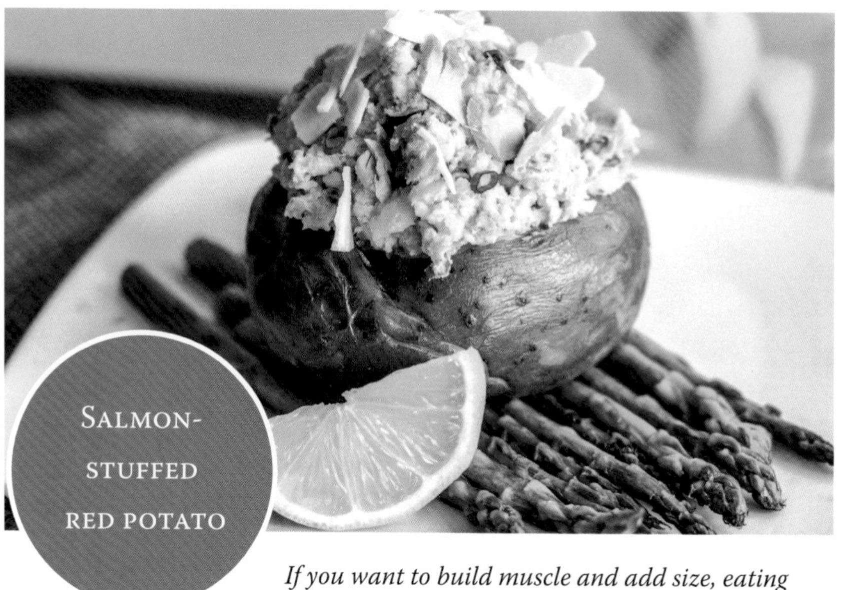

Salmon-stuffed red potato

If you want to build muscle and add size, eating salmon and potatoes is the way to go. Adding salmon is a great way to "dress up" a staple bodybuilding food and turn it into a meal that even a family of picky eaters will enjoy.

Ingredients

6 oz wild salmon (measured raw)

~240g red potato (baked)

1/8 cup 2% Greek yogurt

1 tbsp parmesan

1/4 cup green onion

1 cup grilled asparagus

Seasoning

pepper, coconut aminos, Mrs. Dash chipotle, garlic (optional)

STEPS

Set oven to 375°F.

Bake a red potato until soft.

Season wild salmon with 1 tbsp coconut aminos, pepper, and Mrs. Dash chipotle seasoning.

Bake salmon in the oven for about 10 minutes until finished. Then flake the salmon with a fork and set it aside.

Once the potato is finished, slice it down the middle and remove the insides with a spoon. Place the contents in a bowl.

Mix the potato contents with Greek yogurt, green onion, and fresh garlic. Keep stirring until the contents are creamy.

Add salmon to the mixture and blend with a fork. Season with sea salt to taste.

Top with parmesan cheese (if desired) and enjoy!

Macronutrients | 466 calories, 46g protein, 42g carbs, 14g fat

DAY 2
Take the Step

Step by step

and the thing is

DONE.

—*Charles Atlas*

On December 1, 1955, when Rosa Parks took that remarkably courageous step and refused to move to the back of the bus after a white man got on board and demanded her seat, the city of Montgomery, Alabama, would never be the same, and neither would the United States. That determined step of one humble little seamstress with the heart of a lioness started the American Civil Rights Movement. When she took another step and appealed her conviction during the bus boycott that followed her arrest and conviction, the U.S. Supreme Court would eventually rule that segregation on buses was unconstitutional.

Whether it's changing your physique or changing a nation, it all starts with one step followed by another. Rosa said her mother believed "you should take advantage of the opportunities, no matter how few they were." Rosa stepped across the threshold of her fears, took advantage of her one opportunity, and one day became the first woman to receive the Martin Luther King Nonviolent Peace Prize. Whatever it is that you want to change, take the first step.

What step will you take to change what needs to change in your life?

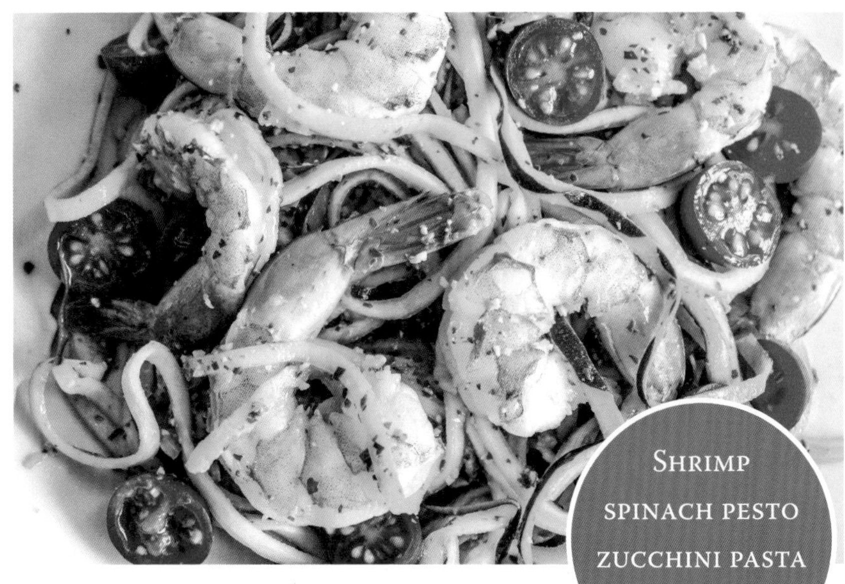

Shrimp spinach pesto zucchini pasta

| 6-8 servings |

Let's face it: "low-carb" days (where you are not eating many carbohydrates) can be not so fun . . . but you can still eat BIG while enjoying a delicious, nutritious, and very filling meal.

Pesto sauce is easy to make and customize for you to use throughout the week. Use wisely: it's delicious so you can get carried away if you are not careful.

Ingredients

1.5 cups basil leaves
1 cup spinach
1/4 cup walnuts
1/3 cup extra virgin olive oil
1/8 cup parmesan
1 garlic clove
Juice from 1 lemon
Peeled and deveined shrimp
Cherry tomatoes
Sea salt

Utensil

Spiralizer

STEPS

Blend basil, spinach, garlic, walnuts, lemon juice, and parmesan in a food processor or blender.

Add olive oil and salt to food processor/blender and continue to blend until smooth.

In a bowl, julienne raw zucchini linguine with spiralizer.

Add pesto sauce to zucchini linguine and mix.

Top with shrimp and cherry tomatoes.

To reduce the amount of calories even more, use less olive oil and add water to the mixture.

Macronutrients per tbsp sauce | 110 calories, 1g protein, 1g carbs, 12g fat

DAY 3
Overcome

Your passion
will not die,
if your
COMMITMENT
does not end.

No matter how hard I've tried to avoid it, I've learned that with passion comes pain, because the disappointment of not achieving your goal(s) can be overwhelming.

Admittedly, in some areas of my life I have allowed the "pain" of not succeeding to cause the fire of my passion to fizzle out. Know what I mean? You didn't win the competition or get the job. Your physique still "looks" the same. He or she said, "Sorry, I'm not ready yet." The list of disappointments grows, and ultimately you just stop "dreaming."

But I'm learning that disappointment is part of the journey. It is not just about winning as much as it is about overcoming. And my dreams can become reality if I just stay committed.

How do you stay focused on accomplishing your goals?

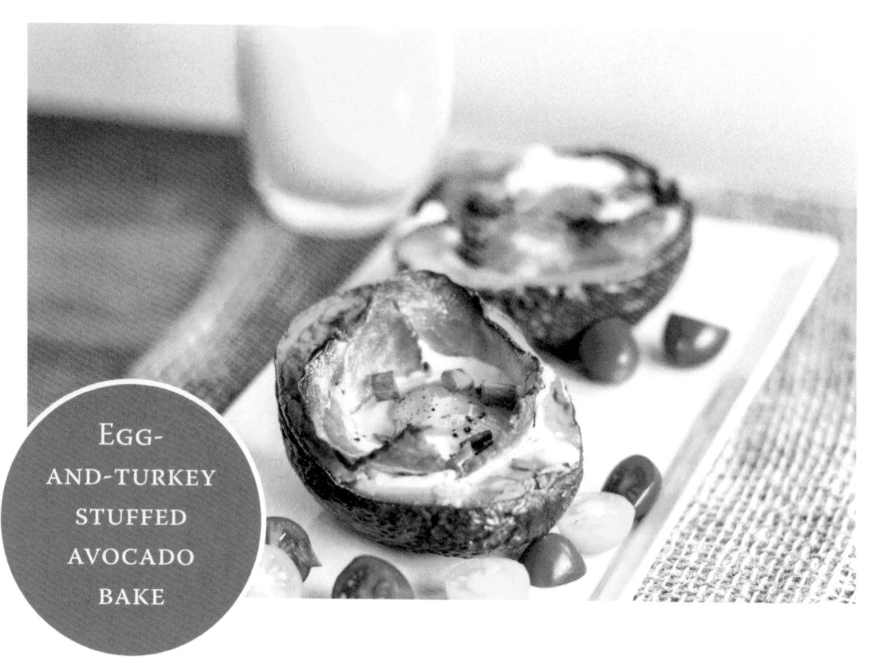

Egg-and-Turkey Stuffed Avocado Bake

Supplying your body with heart healthy fats in the morning can give you energy to conquer your day and power through any morning workout.

Ingredients

1 Haas avocado

2 eggs

2 slices uncured, nitrate-free, natural turkey bacon (or you can use thick turkey leg lunch meat)

STEPS

Set oven to 405°F.

Slice an avocado in half and scoop out part of the insides to make a larger hole.

Create a ring inside of the hole with a piece of turkey bacon.

Crack eggs in a bowl.

Use aluminum foil to form a ring to prop up the avocado halves on a baking sheet so they do not roll from side to side.

Scoop 1 egg yolk out of the bowl using a spoon and place in each of the avocado halves inside of the ring you created with the turkey bacon. Then pour the egg white evenly between the halves. Season if desired with pepper, red pepper, cumin, and a small pinch of sea salt.

Bake in the oven for 22–25 minutes.

Macronutrients for 1/2 turkey & egg baked avocado | 240 calories, 15g protein, 6g carbs, 17g fat

DAY 4
Tap Your Potential

Train your mind to see

PROMISE

and

POTENTIAL

in every situation.

When did we start to settle for "I'm getting by" or "I'm okay at it"? Certainly we all have some limitations, but we all have within us the promise and potential to be extraordinary if we choose to be. Sometime around 350 B.C. the Greek philosopher Aristotle suggested that every person is born with an exclusive set of potentials that yearn to be fulfilled in whatever situations we find ourselves in. But it requires thinking and hoping and praying and wise planning with both eyes open.

You were born with incredible potential, possibilities, creativity, and dreams. You have the abilities and the talents to excel and succeed at becoming what you were created to be. But you have to start tapping into them, and you have to be brave and tap into the situations in front of you that bring new opportunities. Work hard, be determined, and refuse to give up. If you are persistent and prune away whatever tries to create diversions and entanglements, you will get to where you want to be.

Describe the potential you see in one situation in your life today.

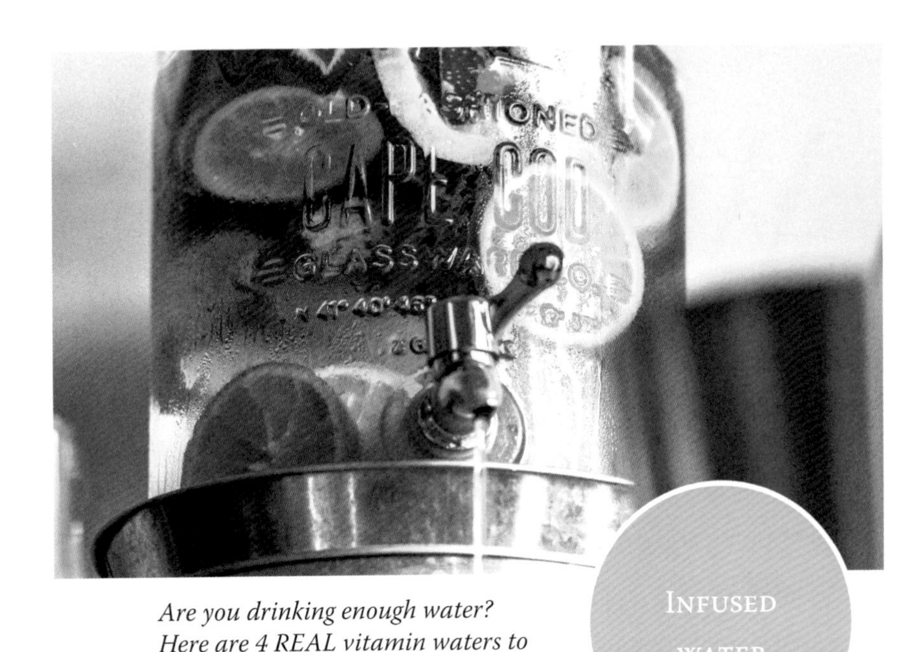

Infused water

*Are you drinking enough water?
Here are 4 REAL vitamin waters to
help with detox, hydration, and energy!*

Ingredients

Orange blueberry water

Benefits | Vitamins C and B6, antioxidants and flavonoids

Cucumber, lime, and mint

Benefits | Great for digestion, appetite control, bloating, vitamins C, A, and K, iron, and calcium

Watermelon, cucumber, and rosemary

Benefits | Reduces bloating, immune defense, vitamins C, A, and B6, and appetite control

Strawberries and lemon

Benefits | Vitamin C, digestion, blood sugar stabilizer, and immune defense

Tips | *Water is best at room temperature. Put as much fruit in the water as you like. Let the water sit for at least 30 minutes before drinking, and sip throughout the day. You can refill your water bottle after you drink it. After 24 hours, you should discard the fruit and make a fresh batch of water. Stay thirsty, my friends!*

168 calories, 19g protein, 15g carbs, 4g fat, 3g fiber

They may criticize
your choices now,
but will seek
your advice later.

STAY
FOCUSED.

I'll never forget the day I stopped my gym workout for 23 minutes to try to explain to a guy why I did not enjoy drinking chocolate milk after workouts. He cited numerous studies about the many benefits, which didn't matter to me because I was following a regimen that seemed to be working for me. Ever been there?

Not everyone will accept your new lifestyle or agree with your choices. Furthermore, there are several healthy ways to achieve the same goal. Spending time defending your healthy choices and lifestyle is not going to get you any closer to achieving your goals. And if you're like me, it can ruin a good workout!

Continue to be humble enough to take criticism and advice, yet wise enough to know when people are just being negative and you need to just be quiet. The best response is sometimes no response at all.

The same people who may talk about you now, may be seeking your advice later. Stay focused, stay encouraged, and stay humble.

How do you handle negative feedback?

....

....

....

....

....

....

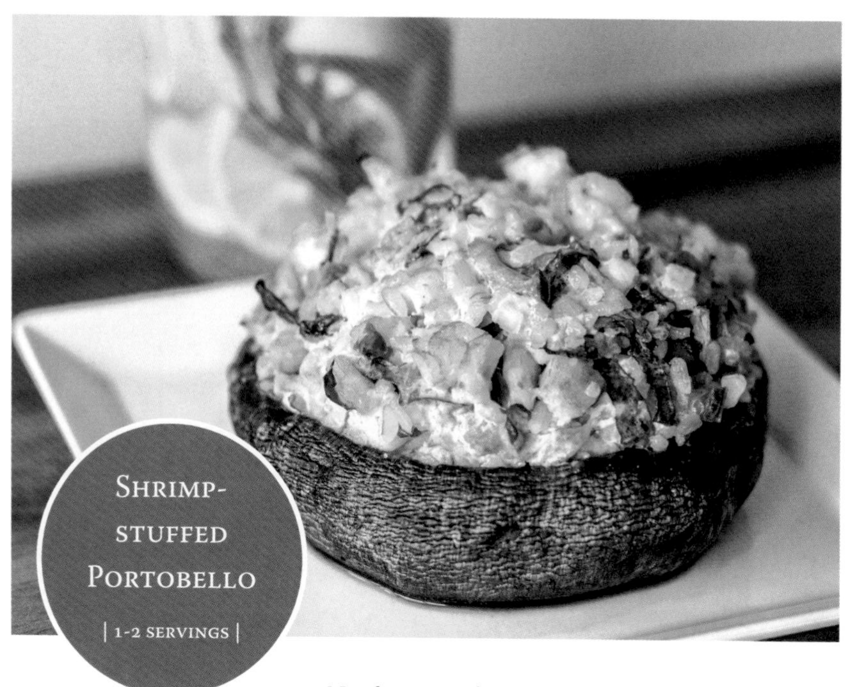

Shrimp-stuffed Portobello

| 1-2 servings |

Need a great dinner idea? Try this recipe. Simple, delicious, and filling! Very easy to customize as well and use different protein sources. Vegans and vegetarians can substitute shrimp for eggplant, zucchini, or tempeh and use quinoa instead of brown rice. Boom!

Ingredients

- 6 oz cooked and chopped shrimp (boiled or in skillet)
- 2 Portobello mushroom caps
- 1 cup cooked brown rice
- 1 cup kale
- 2/3 cup pico de gallo
- 1 oz goat cheese
- 1/3 cup 2% Greek yogurt
- 1/4 cup bell pepper pieces

STEPS

Set the oven to 375°F.

Cook shrimp in skillet or boil.

Once shrimp is cooked, mix in brown rice, kale, pico de gallo, Greek yogurt, and goat cheese.

Remove inside of mushroom caps using a spoon.

Stuff mushroom with mixture.

Bake for 25 minutes at 375°F.

Enjoy!

Macronutrients per serving | 288 calories, 27g protein, 27g carbs, 5g fat

DAY 6
PUSH FORWARD

STRENGTH

doesn't come from

what you can do.

It comes from overcoming the things you thought you couldn't.

—*Ashley Greene*

Strength. What is the first thing that comes to your mind? Olympic strength athletes? Bodybuilders? NFL linemen? Or is it the single mom who is making the extraordinary sacrifices to give her children a good home? Or the child born with a congenital disability who won't stop trying to overcome his or her syndrome?

So are you allowing your weaknesses and insecurities to keep you from being your best? You may not feel capable in your own strength, but that's okay. Our strength to overcome is found in pressing forward through those feelings. Don't focus on your weaknesses; focus on making use of whatever gifts and abilities you have and being the best you can possibly be with them.

Few things in life happen as swiftly as we may like them to, especially success. Keep pushing, fight through the challenges and pain, and become your own personal best. And you may just find yourself using this strength to help strengthen others!

Where do you need to keep pushing forward until you overcome?

....

....

....

....

....

....

....

....

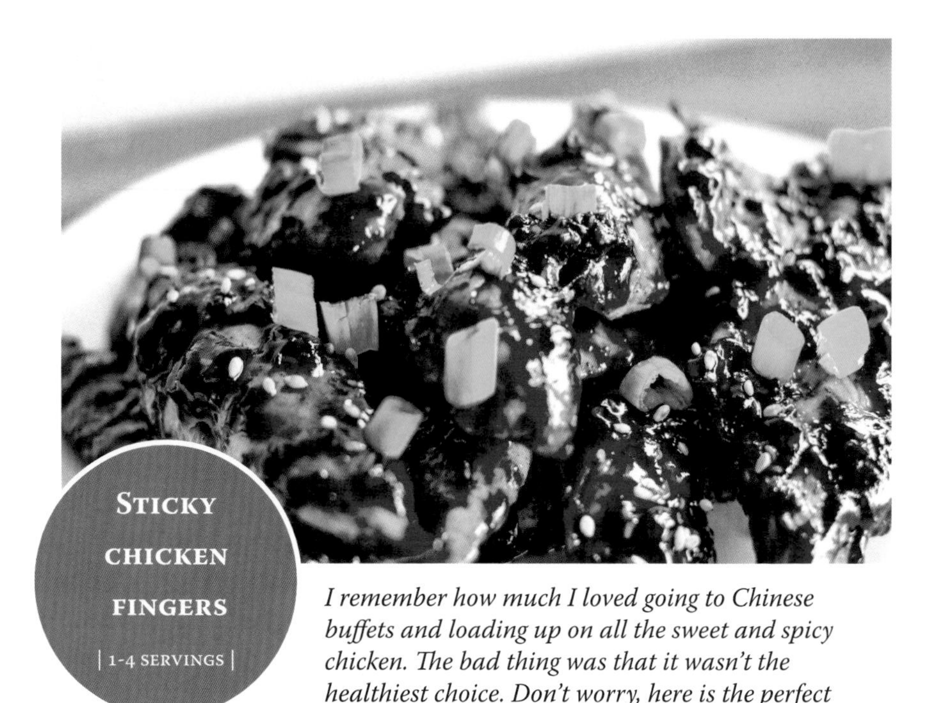

Sticky Chicken Fingers

| 1-4 servings |

I remember how much I loved going to Chinese buffets and loading up on all the sweet and spicy chicken. The bad thing was that it wasn't the healthiest choice. Don't worry, here is the perfect dish to satisfy those cravings for Chinese food for you and your family. Enjoy!

Ingredients

1.25 lb lean chicken tenders (raw)

3/4 cup raspberries

1/4 cup organic raw honey

1/8 cup hoisin

1 tbsp coconut oil

2 tbsp minced garlic

Seasonings

paprika

red pepper flakes

STEPS

Mash raspberries in a bowl.

Sauté garlic in coconut oil. Then add raspberries, hoisin sauce, and finally honey.

Stir and simmer for 5 minutes. Then let it cool in order to thicken.

Dry chicken tenders on a paper towel.

Preheat oven to 375°F.

Place chicken on an oven pan (cover with aluminum paper to prevent mess).

Coat chicken with sauce and rub on all sides. Sprinkle paprika and red pepper flakes.

Bake for 15 minutes at 375°F.

Take out of oven and rub remaining sauce on the chicken.

Devour!

Macronutrients per 1 serving | 254 calories, 27g protein, 23g carbs, 6g fat

DAY 7
Priceless Treasure

TAKE CARE

of your body;

it's the only place

you have to live.

—Jim Rohn

Your body may have its share of imperfections, but you're wise if you take care of it as you would a priceless treasure. For all that it may lack, it is the temple that houses all that you are. It gives you the ability to think and feel and enjoy, and without it you aren't going anywhere.

It has been estimated 80 percent of diseases, such as heart disease, cancer, and type 2 diabetes, are caused by the poor lifestyle choices we make every day, which are correctable. Most people go through life not taking any responsibility for their health. They shuffle along until something goes wrong, then race to the doctor to get it fixed. They take better care of their car than their body.

So what are you doing, now, today? Are you making time for exercise, working on keeping your muscles and bones strong? If not, take those good intentions and start today. Oh, and sleep well, eat healthy and enjoy your food, slow down and live life to the fullest, and listen to what your body is telling you if there is pain. Your body is more important than your car!

So what are you doing, now, today, to care for your body?

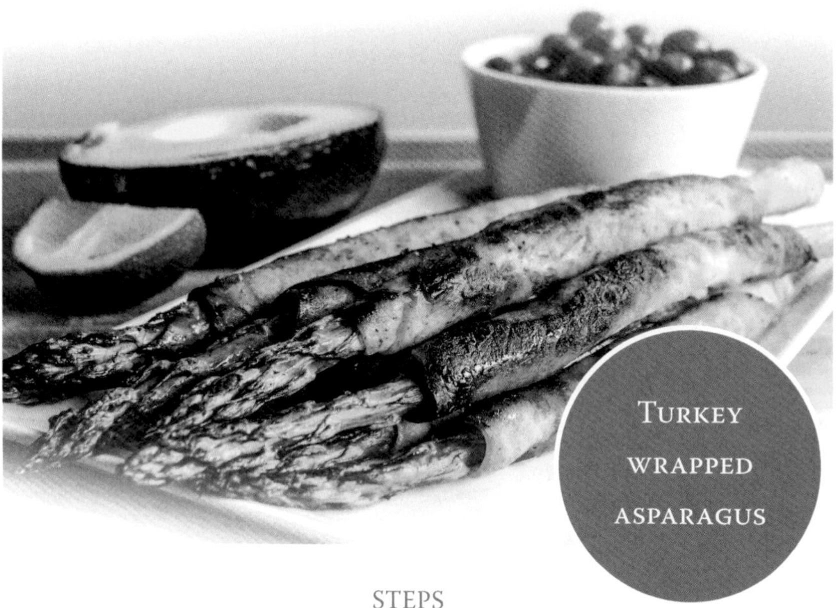

Turkey wrapped asparagus

Ingredients

Low sodium turkey lunch meat

Raw asparagus spears

Choice of seasonings (garlic, cumin, cayenne pepper, pepper)

STEPS

Set oven to broil temperature.

Wash asparagus and cut off bottom stems.

Take 1 slice of low sodium turkey lunch meat and wrap around the asparagus.

Season the asparagus wraps.

Spray a skillet with coconut oil and set on medium-high heat. Allow the skillet to get hot.

Add asparagus to the skillet. Move the skillet around to "roll" the asparagus so that all sides are seared. About 3–5 minutes.

Remove the asparagus from the skillet and place on a baking sheet.

Place in the oven for 4–5 minutes.

Remove and enjoy!

Macronutrients per 6 oz turkey and 8 spears | 176 calories, 36g protein, 5g carbs, 3g fat

WEEK 4 WRAP

1. What recipes did you try this week?

2. What did you like about the recipes?

3. What would you change next time?

4. Which natural fruit and vegetable smoothies did you try?

5. What new power food or complex carb did you research and prepare this week?

6. How much water were you able to drink daily this week?

» Weekly Challenge Checklist

Completed daily devotionals?	
Prepared 5 recipes from Week 1–4?	
Made 2 natural fruit and veggie smoothies?	
Selected one power food or complex carb and prepared it?	
Increased your daily water consumption?	
Extra recipes created?	
Total challenges completed	

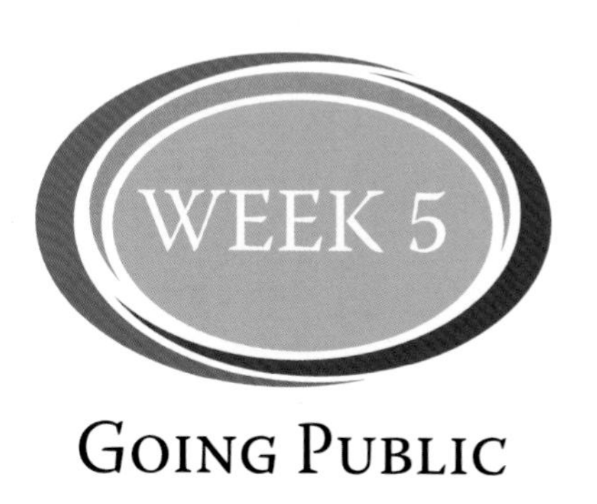

Going Public

Challenges:

- Spend at least 10 minutes to complete the daily devotional.
- Select 5 recipes from Week 1 through Week 5 and prepare them.
- Prepare your lunch or a healthy snack meal every day this week.
- Prepare one of your new favorite healthy meals for someone else, or share something you have learned with someone you trust.
- Remember to adjust all recipes and portion sizes to complement your dietary needs and fitness goals.

DAY 1
Be Strong

SUCCESS

often invites scorn.

Here's a modern-day translation: "Haters are going to hate." So, are you strong enough to handle success?

I often receive messages from people who have lost weight saying that their friends or family treat them differently. Some make negative comments about their physique or lifestyle that can be discouraging. And this is certainly not limited to fitness. In any scenario, the idea that your loved ones will criticize your good intentions can "knock the wind" out of almost anyone.

I've realized that success is often met with negativity that is masked as "disbelief."

It is disbelief that the change you experienced in your life can actually happen for them. So instead of being defensive, recognize it for what it really is—just another opinion. Stay true to yourself and keep it moving! Be humble, realizing that change may not come as easy for others. Yet stay hungry so you keep on progressing. Let the haters do what they do best—talk.

What "talk" are you hearing that you need to disregard?

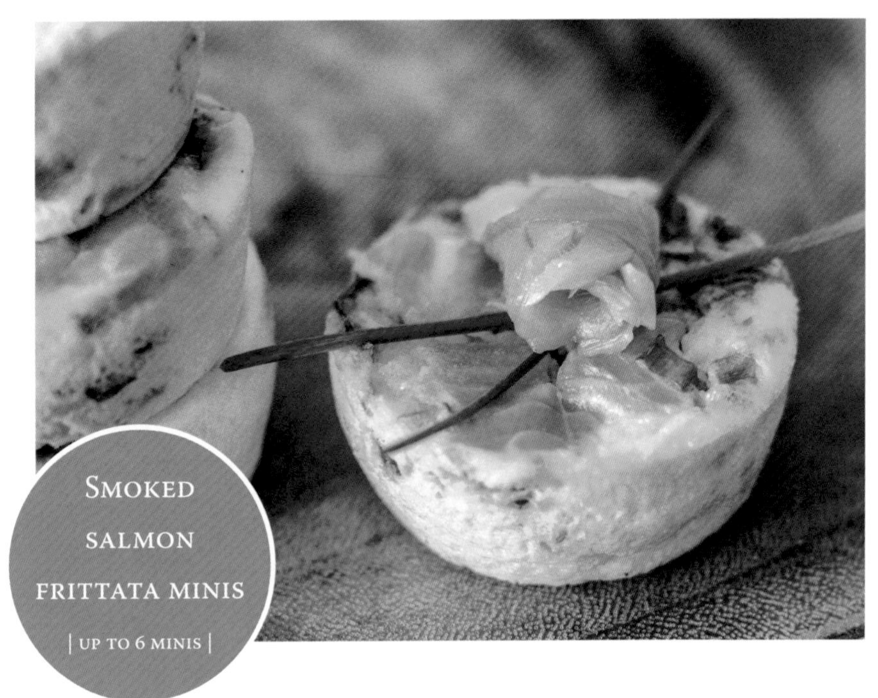

Smoked salmon frittata minis

| up to 6 minis |

Ingredients

2 eggs

4 egg whites

1/3 cup plain Greek yogurt

4 oz smoked salmon

1/4 cup goat cheese crumble

1 cup chopped arugula (or spinach)

1/8 cup chopped green onions

Seasonings

red pepper, pepper to taste

STEPS

Set the oven to 350°F.

In bowl, whisk eggs with Greek yogurt.

Add green onions, salmon, goat cheese, and arugula to the bowl and mix with a spatula. If desired, add red pepper and/or pepper. Remember that smoked salmon tends to be high in sodium, so I do not advise adding any seasoning that contains sodium.

Spray muffin cups with coconut oil and pour in the mixture.

Bake for 20 minutes at 350°F or until the egg is completely cooked.

Enjoy!

Macronutrients per frittata mini | 103 calories, 12g protein, 1g carb, 5g fat

DAY 2
Break Mental Barriers

Your fitness

is 100% mental.

Your body won't go
where your mind doesn't
PUSH IT.

—Heather Frey

Did you know that for the longest time, track-and-field experts were emphatic that it was impossible for a runner to break the four-minute-mile barrier. But one day in the early 1950s, a young man named Roger Bannister began to train, believing he could do the "impossible." When he broke the four-minute-mile barrier, it was called the "Miracle Mile." So what? Well, after no one had ever done it before, within the next ten years, 336 more runners also did it! After all those years, Bannister proved it was a mental barrier, not a physical one.

Most of us have a mental barrier when it comes to personal fitness. The body begins to do its part, but the brain starts screaming that you'll never succeed getting yourself into shape. You're too weak, too overweight, and too busy, right? Wrong! You have the strength and what you need to keep moving forward, but you have to tell yourself the truth and break the mental barrier. Start thinking and believing positively. Your "Miracle Mile" is possible!

What mental barrier do you have that limits your fitness?

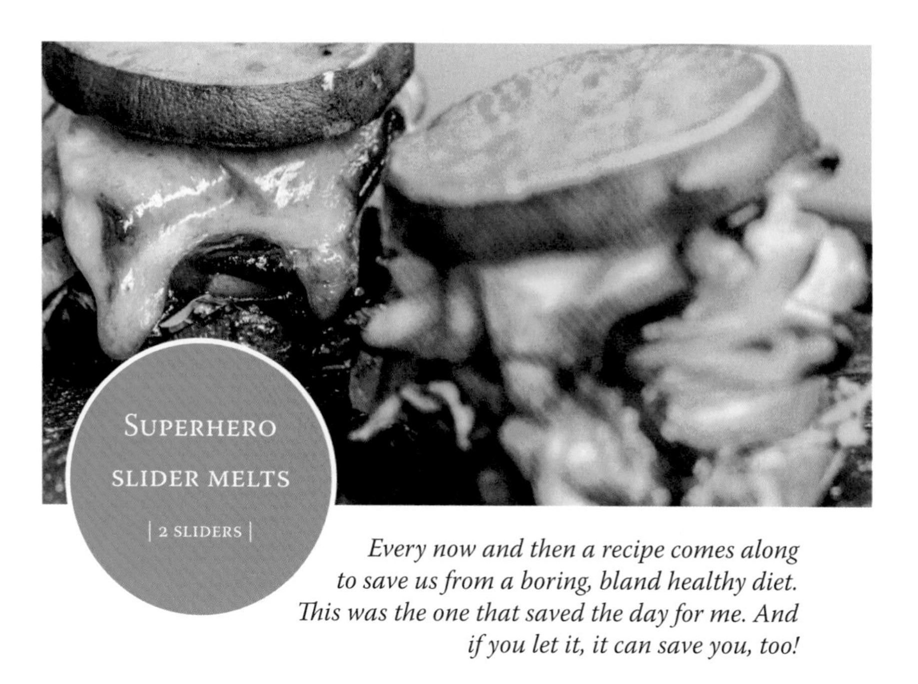

Superhero slider melts

| 2 sliders |

Every now and then a recipe comes along to save us from a boring, bland healthy diet. This was the one that saved the day for me. And if you let it, it can save you, too!

Ingredients

200g (4 x 50g) sweet potato cut into thick pieces

6 oz turkey lunch meat

1 slice mozzarella cheese

Small handful of spinach

2 Roma tomato slices

2 tsp BBQ sauce

STEPS

Set oven to 375°F.

Slice a sweet potato into 4 thick pieces to make the buns of the sliders.

Cut the slice of mozzarella cheese into 4 pieces.

On one sweet potato slice, add spinach, 1 tomato slice, 3 oz turkey meat, 2 mozzarella cheese pieces, and 1 tsp BBQ sauce.

Top with the other sweet potato slice and jam a wooden kabob skewer all the way through the entire slider so that it pierces the sweet bun below.

Repeat for the other slider.

Place them on a baking sheet and bake for 30 minutes at 375°F or until the sweet potato is cooked to desired firmness/softness. I prefer them to be firm so that you can hold it like a slider.

Allow the sliders to cool before eating.

Macronutrients per slider | 239 calories, 24g protein, 23g carbs, 4g fat

DAY 3
Confront It

The heaviest
WEIGHT
you will ever lift
is the problem you
refuse to
CONFRONT.

I got punched in the stomach by a friend the other day—never saw it coming. I was helping him out with some diet and fitness related guidance when he said, "Hey, so I see you've been working out a lot recently. You're looking good." Then he paused for a moment and said, "Man, I love you when I say this, but don't use this fitness and nutrition stuff as a way to avoid what's really going on here. You still need to get back out there and find someone. You can't stay single."

I'm not going to lie—that hurt. But it was the truth. It made me realize how easy it is to get so "busy with life" that you don't have to confront problems that really challenge and stretch you. While I'll never give up fitness and this healthier lifestyle, I realized the need to deal with problems before they get "heavier."

What's your heavy weight to deal with?

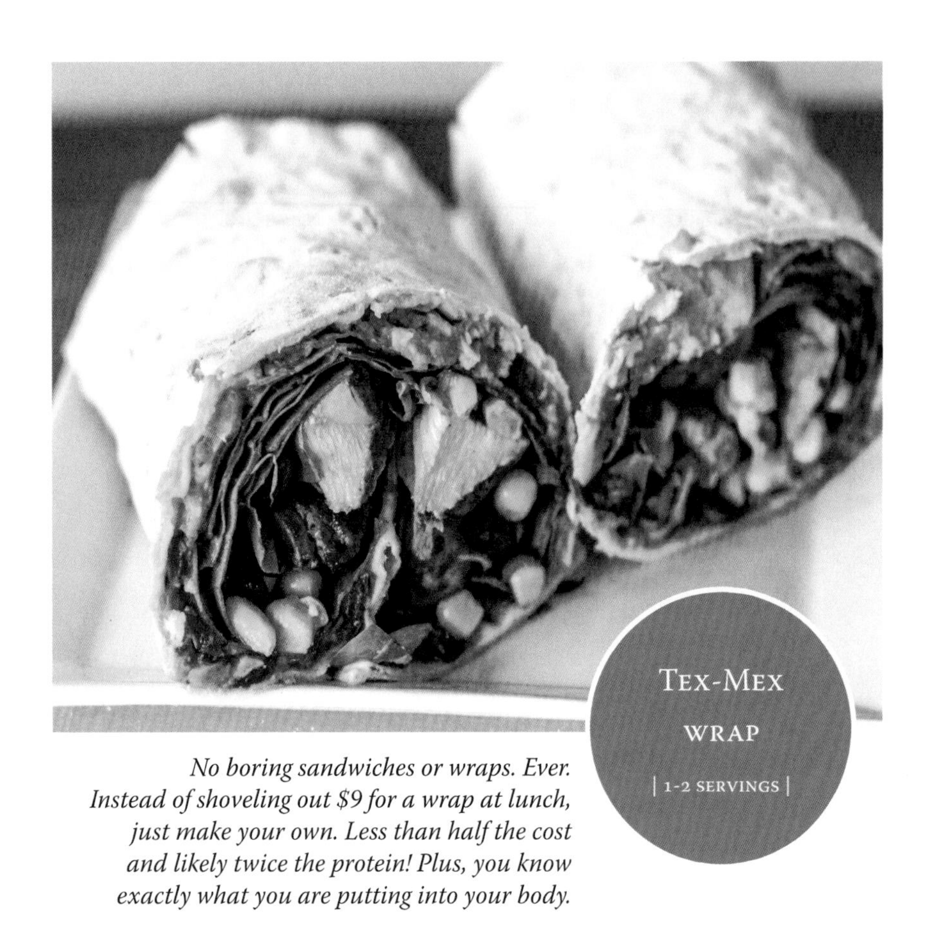

Tex-Mex Wrap

| 1-2 servings |

No boring sandwiches or wraps. Ever. Instead of shoveling out $9 for a wrap at lunch, just make your own. Less than half the cost and likely twice the protein! Plus, you know exactly what you are putting into your body.

Ingredients

6 oz chicken breast

1 wheat lavash bread (flat bread)

1/3 Haas avocado

2 tbsp pico de gallo

Handful spinach

2 tbsp black beans

2 tbsp corn

Seasonings for chicken

Bragg's Liquid Aminos (or sea salt), Mrs. Dash Chipotle

STEPS

Season chicken breast. Cook in a nonstick skillet on medium-high heat.

Cube or slice the chicken breast into strips.

In a bowl, mix avocado with pico de gallo.

Spread avocado mix on lavash bread.

Add spinach, corn, black beans, and chicken.

Roll up the lavash bread, cut in half, and enjoy!

Macronutrients for one serving | 456 calories, 44g protein, 42g carbs, 12g fat

DAY 4
Age Means… Nothing

It's never too late to

BECOME

what you might

have been.

—George Eliot

You don't have to be sixty or eighty years old to find yourself stuck in the quagmire of "should haves, could haves, would haves," and to believe that it's too late to follow your heart. As a 31-year-old single mom on welfare, J. K. Rowling must have surely had huge doubts as to whether she'd ever have a shot at being published. Harrison Ford was pounding nails as a carpenter till in his 30s. What was going through his head as the clock ticked? McDonald's founder Ray Kroc sold paper cups and milkshake mixers till he was 52. Arianna Huffington started the *Huffington Post* at the age of 54.

It doesn't matter what your age is. You can be twenty and yet feel "too old" because you're allowing other people to control you and determine your future. It's a certain recipe for an unfulfilled and frustrated life. Whatever your age, shake off the regrets of yesterday and yesteryear and start with a new vision of who you can become. That's actually good advice for every day!

Where do you feel it's too late for you? What is the truth you need to tell yourself?

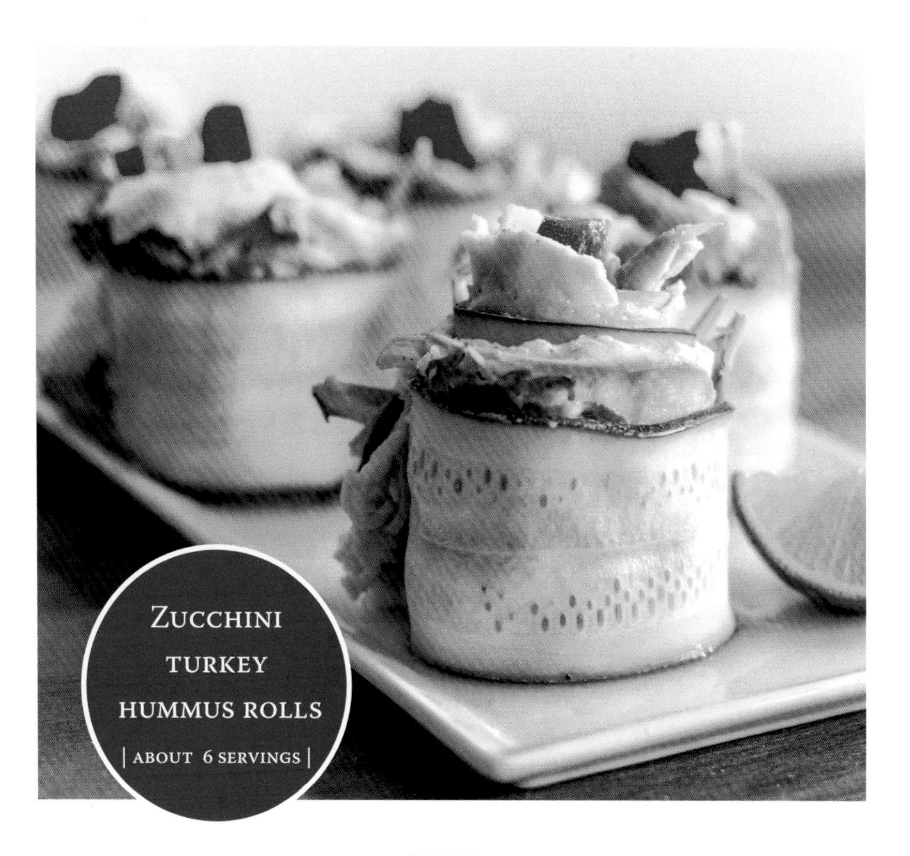

Zucchini turkey hummus rolls

| about 6 servings |

Ingredients

3/4 zucchini

4 tbsp hummus

8 oz low sodium turkey lunch meat

1/4 cup feta crumble (optional)

1 jalapeño

Utensil

Mandolin

STEPS

Slice zucchini in long strips with mandolin or a really sharp knife.

On each piece of zucchini, spread about 1 tsp of hummus.

Slice jalapeño and add 2 slices to one end of the zucchini piece.

Add just a little bit of feta crumble to the roll.

Place 2 pieces of folded turkey along the length of the zucchini.

Roll the zucchini up and secure it with a toothpick.

Repeat for each roll.

Macronutrients per roll without feta | 70 calories, 9g protein, 4g carbs, 2g fat

Learn to love
YOURSELF
FIRST.

*Stop waiting for
others to love you.*

Sometimes I ask myself, "Do I really love me?" Admittedly, I surprised myself when the question first popped in my head. With all the exercising and nutrition and activities I do, I question whether I am really doing it for me, or for the recognition and approval of others (or that special someone)? Eh, maybe it's a little of both.

I constantly have to remind myself on my journey of life to be comfortable with me—imperfections and all—and to not lose myself in all the change.

So what I see is what I get. I am what I am, and that's who I need to love.

So do you really love yourself? Truly?

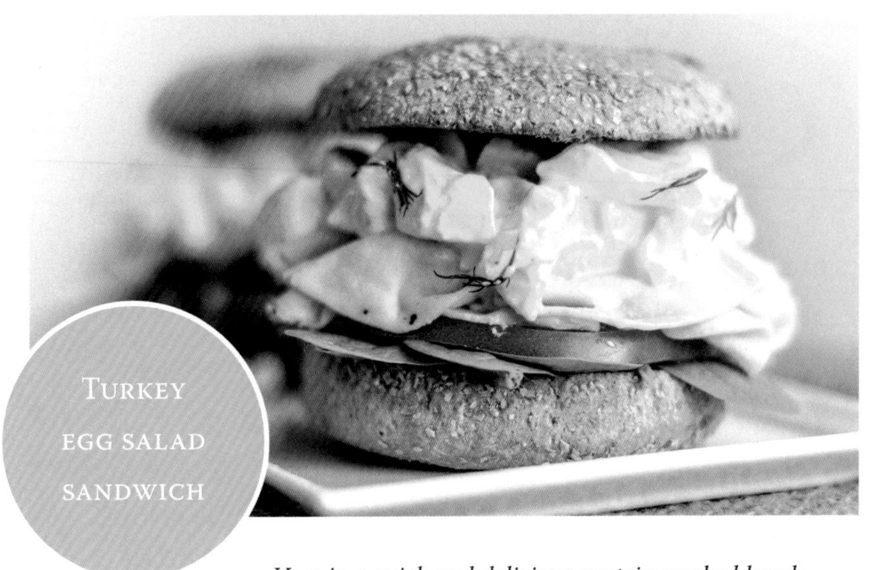

Turkey egg salad sandwich

Here is a quick and delicious protein-packed lunch you will most definitely enjoy! Plus, it's an easy way to get rid of some of the lean leftover turkey or lunch meat from the week.

Ingredients

1 whole grain bun

2 oz turkey lunch meat or turkey breast (shredded)

1 egg

3 egg whites

1/4 cup Greek yogurt

1/2 tbsp mustard (recommend a spicy mustard like Dijon)

Fresh spinach and tomato for the sandwich

Seasonings

garlic (minced or powder), fresh dill, sea salt and pepper to taste, spinach, tomato

STEPS

Boil eggs. Once finished, peel eggs and place in a bowl.

Remove the egg yolk from 3 of the eggs and discard. Leave the other yolk.

Chop eggs into tiny pieces and place in a bowl.

Add yogurt, mustard, and seasonings to the bowl. Mix together using a fork.

Build your sandwich. Add spinach, tomato, turkey, and then the egg salad.

Macronutrients per sandwich | 378 calories, 45g protein, 30g carbs, 8g fat

DAY 6
Work for It

If you can't stop thinking about it,
don't stop
WORKING
for it.

—Author Unknown

Thomas Edison had to be one of the coolest, most amazing nerds who ever lived. He once said, "I speak without exaggeration when I say that I have constructed 3,000 different theories in connection with the electric light, each one of them reasonable and apparently likely to be true. Yet in two cases only did my experiments prove the truth of my theory." He couldn't stop thinking about inventing the light bulb, and he didn't stopped working for it until he got it.

Edison did extraordinary things because he first believed and then he took a step of faith. And the same is true for us. If you have a dream that has captured your heart and mind, go for it. So what if it takes 3,000 attempts to turn it into reality. You can't play it safe if you want to realize the fulfillment of your dream. Step out, step up, and be willing to find out what you really can do with your gifts and talents.

Where do you need to stop playing it safe and holding back?

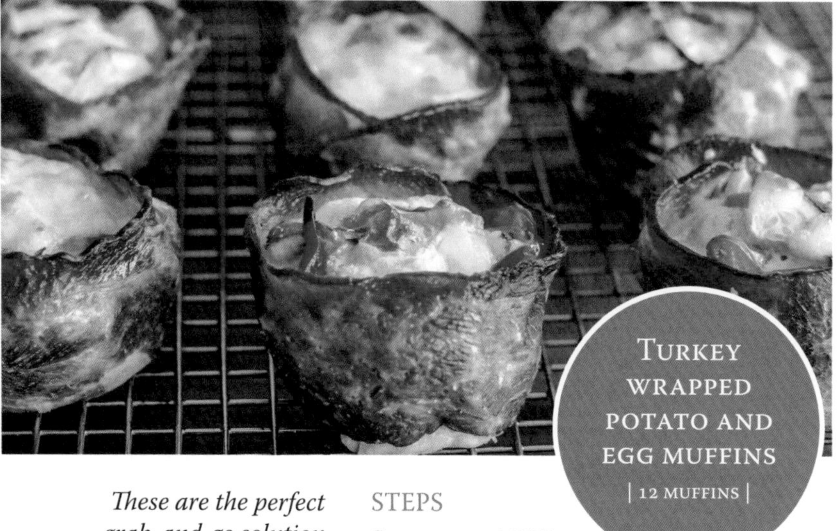

Turkey wrapped potato and egg muffins

| 12 MUFFINS |

These are the perfect grab-and-go solution for busy mornings.

Ingredients

12 slices turkey bacon (natural, uncured, nitrate free, turkey leg meat)

4 eggs

6 egg whites

500g red potato (measured uncooked)

3/4 cup mozzarella cheese

1/2 large zucchini (chopped)

2/3 cup (red) bell pepper (chopped)

2/3 red onion (chopped)

Seasonings

garlic powder, sea salt, pepper, cumin (optional)

STEPS

Set oven to 405°F.

Measure out red potato using a food scale, then chop into pieces. Season with garlic, sea salt, and pepper and place on a baking sheet. Bake in the oven for about 20 minutes at 405°F.

Chop up your veggies and set aside.

Beat eggs in a bowl and add mozzarella cheese, then set aside.

Remove red potato pieces from the oven.

Spray a muffin pan with baking spray and add one strip of turkey bacon to a muffin mold to form a ring.

Add a few pieces of baked red potato and then chopped veggies.

Carefully pour the egg and cheese mixture into the muffin molds, covering the potato and chopped veggies.

Bake in the oven for about 35 minutes at 375°F or until the egg is completely cooked.

When they are finished baking, allow them to cool for a few minutes before removing from the mold.

Enjoy them while they are warm. Or place them on a cooling rack or plate to cool to room temperature, then refrigerate and freeze them to eat throughout the week.

Macronutrients per muffin | 127 calories, 14g protein, 8g carbs, 4g fat

DAY 7
Contentment

Two things define you:

your patience when you have nothing and your attitude when you have

EVERYTHING.

—Author Unknown

If you listen to people's conversations, you realize there are a whole lot of folks who think they are not going to be happy until something significant changes in their life. One person is looking for the big salary and a bigger house, another is demanding that their spouse changes, and most think they won't be happy until they get rid of their problems. If that's you—let me tell you from experience—you're deceiving yourself, and you'll end up extremely discontented with all of your life, not just that part.

It's all about attitude.

You can have it all—the money, the fame, the sex, the power, the career, the long list of awards and accomplishments, and whatever else your heart desires—and that doesn't mean you'll feel satisfied or content and be able to enjoy the "things" you've been able to accumulate.

I've realized that true contentment begins with you. When you become happy with you and the progress you are making in life, then finding the "perfect scenario" for happiness is less important, and just enjoying life's moments is everything.

How would you describe your contentment with where you are today?

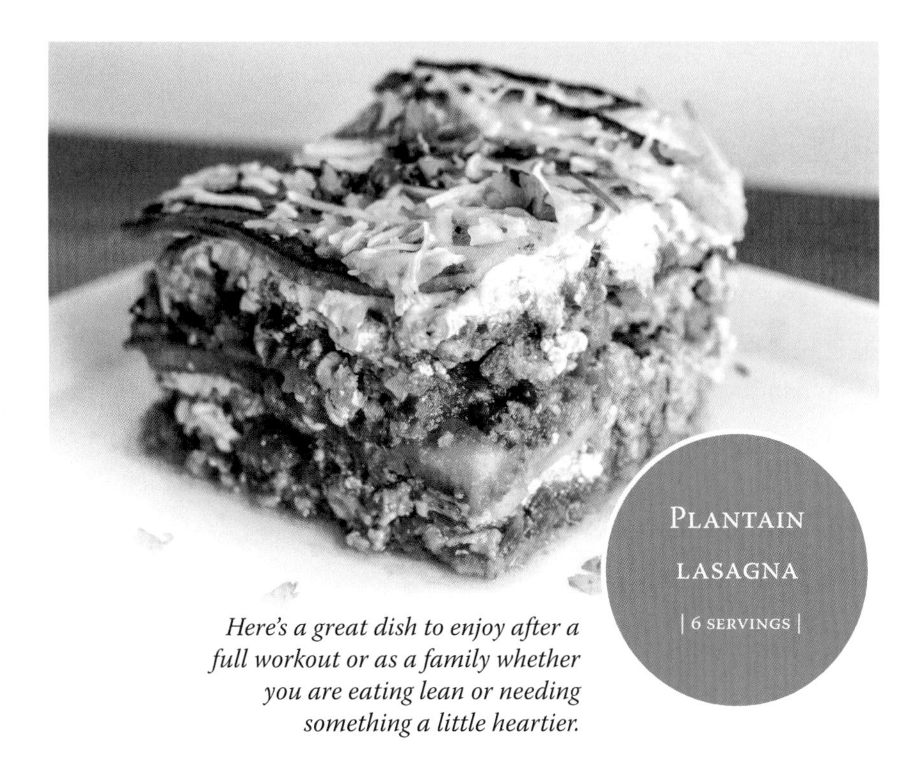

Plantain lasagna

| 6 servings |

Here's a great dish to enjoy after a full workout or as a family whether you are eating lean or needing something a little heartier.

Ingredients

- 1 lb 95% ground turkey
- 2 large ripe plantains (600g)
- 2 cups marinara (low sodium)
- 2 egg whites
- 2/3 cup cottage cheese
- 2 tbsp goat cheese
- 1/3 cup parmesan cheese
- 1/2 cup onions
- 1/3 cup cilantro

Seasoning

cumin, garlic, onion powder, sea salt, and pepper

STEPS

Slice plantains into long pieces.

In a nonstick skillet set to medium-high heat, add 1 tbsp coconut oil, and sear plantains until slightly golden and remove from skillet.

In a bowl, season meat with garlic, cumin, garlic powder, cilantro, onion, pepper, salt, onion powder and mix well.

Cook meat in skillet until brown and add 2 cups of marinara sauce and let simmer.

In a glass casserole dish layer plantain, meat sauce, 1/3 cup cottage cheese, 1 tbsp goat cheese. Repeat this process again.

At the end, pour 2 egg whites over the lasagna. Top with 1/2 cup parmesan cheese.

Cover the dish with foil and bake for 25 minutes at 350°F.

Macronutrients per serving | 561 calories, 44g protein, 59g carbs, 18g fat

WEEK 5 WRAP

1. What recipes did you try this week?

2. What did you like about the recipes?

3. What would you change next time?

4. What lunch or healthy snack meal did you decide to prepare daily?

5. Who did you cook your healthy meal for or share your healthy meal with? How did that feel for you?

» Weekly Challenge Checklist

Completed daily devotionals?	
Prepared 3 recipes from Week 1–5?	
Prepared lunch or healthy snack daily?	
Prepared and shared healthy meal with someone else?	
Extra recipes created?	
Total challenges completed	

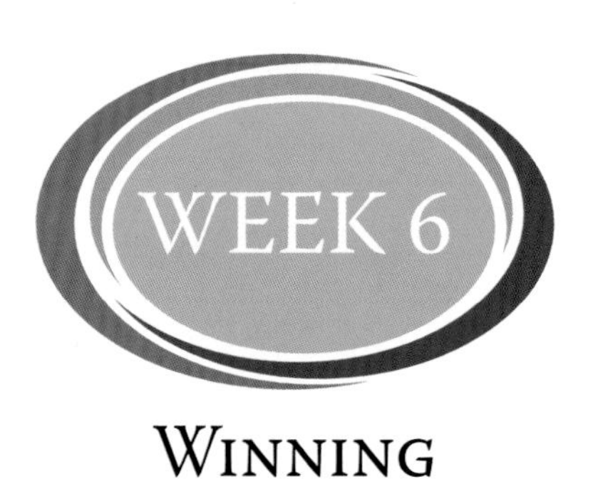

Winning

Challenges:

- Spend at least 10 minutes in the morning to complete the daily devotional.
- Select 5 recipes from Week 1 through Week 6 and prepare them.
- Create your own healthy meal incorporating one lean protein, one complex carbohydrate or power food, and one healthy fat.
- Assess your progress.
- Set a new radical—*yet realistic*—fitness goal and pursue it relentlessly.
- Pay it forward—invest in someone else's fitness journey in small ways, such as paying for a gym membership or purchasing this challenging recipe book for them.
- Remember to adjust all recipes and portion sizes to complement your dietary needs and fitness goals.

DAY 1
Live More

Do work *but*

Do not forget to

LIVE.

When was the last time you enjoyed a night out with friends without having anxiety over your diet? Or how many times have you missed spending time with friends/ family because you opted for a workout or working on projects? If you're like me, the answers are "I can't remember" and "Too many."

I'm learning that building relationships with others is equally as important as staying on track to achieve goals. One night out every once in a while will not hinder you from accomplishing your fitness or career goals.

Life is about creating moments. And that's hard to do when you are alone working in the kitchen, gym, or office.

By all means, attack your goals, but don't let it so completely consume your life that you sacrifice significant opportunities to connect with others. You're so much more than your body and career.

Where do you need to start living more?

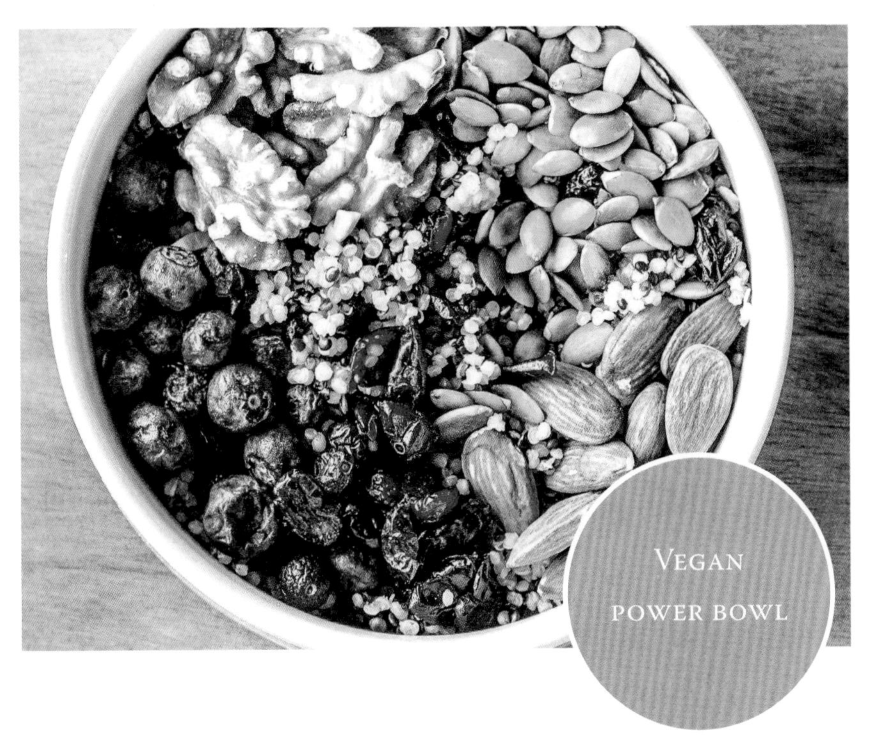

Vegan Power Bowl

This bowl is loaded with natural sugars, protein, and healthy fats to give you energy to power through the day.

Ingredients

2/3 cup cooked quinoa

1 tbsp dried cranberries

1/8 cup blueberries

1 tbsp walnuts

1 tbsp pepitas (or pumpkin seeds)

1 tbsp almonds

1 tsp Maca powder for energy

1/3–1/2 cup almond milk

Cinnamon to taste

STEPS

Cook quinoa using water and allow it to cool to room temperature or store it in the refrigerator for use throughout the week.

In a bowl, add quinoa, then the rest of the ingredients including the Maca powder. If you would like the quinoa to be warm, then heat it in the microwave for a few seconds before adding the ingredients.

Pour almond milk over the quinoa and berry mixture, then sprinkle with a little cinnamon. Stir and enjoy.

Macronutrients | 328 calories, 11g protein, 43g carbs, 16g fat

DAY 2
Stop Running Away

A head full of fears
has no space for
DREAMS.
—*Author Unknown*

Living fearfully, living without confidence, being afraid to step outside the norm, being uptight about change, surrendering to that voice inside our head that says, "That dream of yours, just forget it. You can't do it. You don't have what it takes, and you've proven it over and over in your past flops." Just writing those words is painful, let alone living in such a miserable state.

If you're tired of the torment, first realize that if you don't stop running away from confronting the fear, you'll be running forever. Remember that any fear begins as a thought that then affects your emotions and spreads to your behaviors. If we believe wrong thoughts, we allow ourselves to be ruled by fear, worry, or anxiety—cruel masters. If we change our thinking to the truth and confront the fear head-on, it has to flee, and you'll be free to chase your dreams.

What fear are you prepared to confront with the truth?

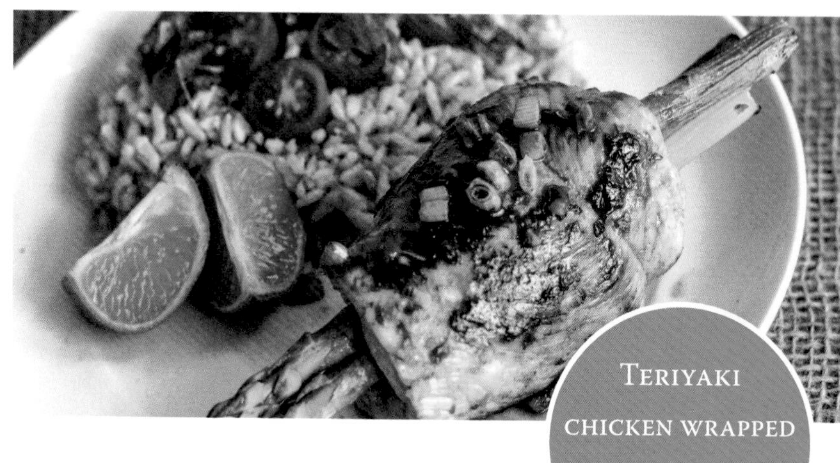

Teriyaki Chicken Wrapped Asparagus

| 2 SERVINGS |

Hands down, this is one of my favorite meals. It's a super easy way to get your daily dose of veggies, and it's easily customizable so you can really make the meal your own.

Ingredients

Two 6 oz chicken breasts thinly sliced

6 thick asparagus spears

Sauce

1 tbsp coconut aminos

1 tbsp raw honey

1 tbsp red chili garlic paste

1 tsp ginger (minced)

1 tsp rice vinegar

1 tsp water

1 green onion chopped

STEPS

Set oven to 375°F.

Cut and trim fat from chicken breast so that it is about 6 oz. If the breast is very thick, pound with your fist or meat mallet to soften and flatten. The meat should be thin enough to roll and close. Set aside in a bowl.

Pour the sauce over the chicken and mix thoroughly, ensuring all sides of the chicken breasts are covered. Refrigerate and marinate for at least 30 minutes. I prefer marinating at least four hours. If you chose to marinate for a long time, be sure to place chicken in an airtight bag or container with the sauce.

Trim the bottom stems from the asparagus spears.

Place three asparagus spears at the thick end of the chicken breast and completely roll the asparagus in chicken.

Place the roll on a baking sheet or foil lined pan with the ending flap down so the chicken roll bakes closed.

Drizzle excess sauce over the chicken roll.

Place foil over the tips of the asparagus spears to prevent any burning during baking.

Bake rolls for 10–12 minutes. If you have extra time before baking, brown all sides of the chicken roll in a nonstick skillet set to medium heat for 3–4 minutes. This will enhance the flavor of your chicken.

Macronutrients per roll | 236 calories, 41g protein, 14g carbs, 4g fat

DAY 3
Faith

Mirrors show you
TODAY.
Faith shows you
TOMORROW.

Looking in the mirror and not seeing what you want can be frustrating, especially when that voice pops into your head and whispers, "This is as good as it gets for you." Aagghh! I hate that voice. I'm sure you've heard the same and more.

Well, in those moments when I'm tempted to lose hope, I remind myself that no matter what my situation looks like, if I can just hold on to fight one more day, I will be closer to achieving my goal.

I know it's tough because you see your present circumstances so clearly in the reflection in the mirror. It can look like change is never going to happen. I'm learning to stop using "the mirror" as my sole compass not only in fitness but also in life. I choose faith.

And while my situation (or physique) may not evolve as quickly as I want it to, I am encouraged that with every step I take by faith, I will get one step closer to realizing my goals. Through faith *and* hard work, my tomorrow seems so much brighter and possible.

How do you motivate yourself to keep going?

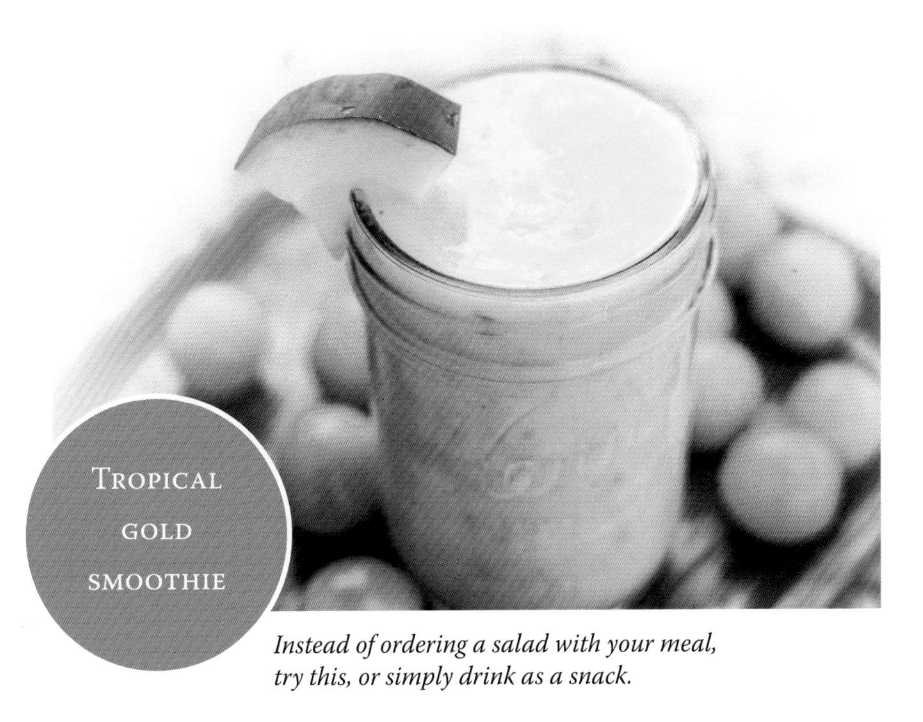

Tropical gold smoothie

Instead of ordering a salad with your meal, try this, or simply drink as a snack.

Ingredients

10 yellow cherry tomatoes

1/2 cup mango (chopped)

1/2 banana

1/4 cup pineapple

1/4 cucumber (peeled)

splash of coconut water (optional)

STEPS

Add ingredients to a blender.

Simply pulse blend for about 1 minute to ensure you remove any chunks, then blend until smooth.

BENEFITS

- Cherry tomatoes contain an antioxidant called lycopene, which has been shown to help lower your risk of cardiovascular disease and even cancer
- Vitamin B-6 has been shown to help the body metabolize protein and help improve brain health
- Supports skin and eye health
- Mangos have pectin, which have been known to help in lowering levels of bad (LDL) cholesterol

Macronutrients (without coconut water) | 173 calories, 3g protein, 43g carbs, 0g fat

DAY 4
Keep Getting Up

You just can't beat the person who
NEVER GIVES UP.

—Babe Ruth

I hope you don't get the idea that I think life is easy. Times are often tough, and I know how discouraged I can get when things do not go my way. The temptation is always right there to give up when the door of opportunity doesn't open or to take the easy way out and just sort of drift along with life's currents when the dream starts to fizzle and sputter. Maybe things don't look as though they'll ever get any better even after you've done everything you know how to do. Nothing's worked.

Perhaps you're on the edge of giving up on something right now. Don't do it! Get back up and keep doing the right thing. Start believing for greater things. It might be for weight loss, for a better marriage, for better health, or for abundance in your life. It might mean to keep believing for a life filled with love, joy, and peace. Focus on your goal, set your course, and don't give up. Keep getting up and you will make it!

Where in your life do you need to get back and start fighting for it?

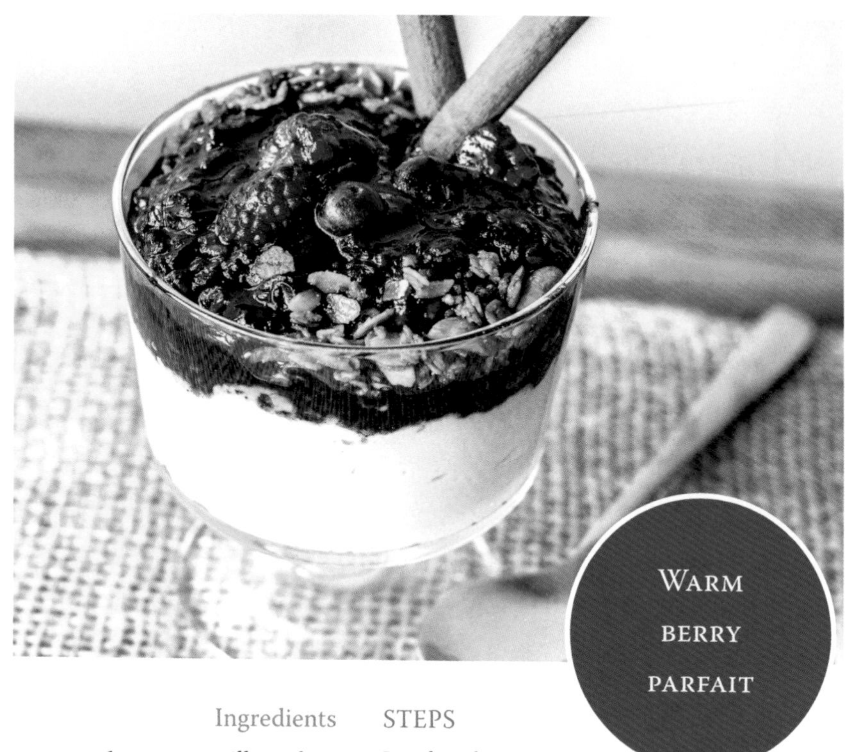

Warm Berry Parfait

Ingredients

1 scoop vanilla isolate whey protein (no carbohydrates, no sugar, no fat)

1/3 cup mixed berries (blueberries, raspberries, blackberries)

1/2 tbsp coconut oil

7 oz Greek yogurt

1/8 cup granola

Spices: cinnamon

STEPS

In a bowl, mix isolate protein powder with Greek yogurt. Add cinnamon and continue to stir until the mixture is smooth and there are no lumps of protein.

Set a nonstick skillet on medium heat and add coconut oil. Add berries to the skillet and stir with a spatula. Allow the berries to "burst" under the heat to create natural, sweet syrup.

Cover the skillet and reduce the heat to low and allow the berries to cook for 2–3 minutes, being careful not to let them burn.

Build the parfait. Add the protein yogurt mixture to a bowl, then add granola on top.

Pour the warm berries over the granola.

Enjoy!

Macronutrients | 419 calories, 46g protein, 24g carbs, 16g fat

DAY 5
Truth Tellers

TRUTH

can set you free,

but first it

will make you mad.

We've all been there. That moment when you go ape on someone, or vice versa, over some feedback. It happened to me early in my fitness journey when my brother advised me to lift lighter weights because my form was terrible. I was angry and insulted at the notion. If I went any lighter, I would have been using the rubber weights from the aerobics class! Okay, maybe not, but he was right about the form.

Maybe for you it's a friend saying, "I thought you were watching what you eat?" Or "Was that the right thing to say?" Or "Maybe that picture you shared on social media was too much?"

We need to deal with the "truths" in our lives that expose what is holding us back from becoming our best. And if people do not accept your advice when you speak the truth, it's cool! Oftentimes it is not your job to convince as much as it is to convey heartfelt truth. Just don't be rude and harsh.

How do you handle receiving "truth"?

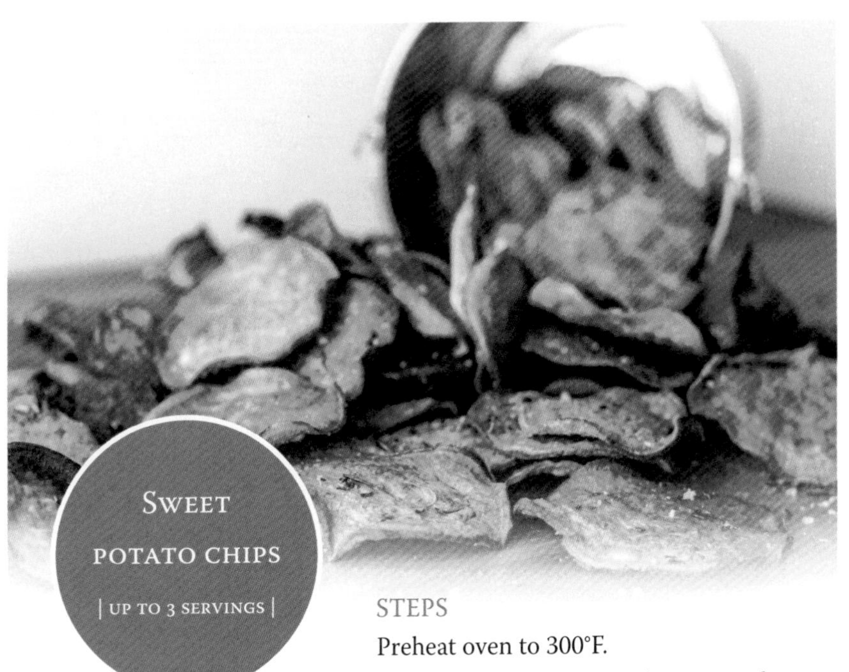

Sweet potato chips

| up to 3 servings |

Ingredients

2 large sweet potatoes (roughly 500g)

coconut oil spray

sea salt

rosemary (fresh, ground)

garlic

Utensils

mandolin (or sharp knife) to cut the potato

wire rack for cooling

STEPS

Preheat oven to 300°F.

Slice a sweet potato into thin 1/8-inch thick pieces using a mandolin or a sharp knife. Keep in mind that chips that are too thick will take longer to bake and may not become crispy.

Line a baking sheet with parchment paper and place the slices on the baking sheet.

Spray the pieces with coconut oil and sprinkle with sea salt and bake for 20 minutes at 300°F.

Remove them from the oven and flip the slices over. Bake for another 20 minutes at 300°F.

Remove the chips and check for flimsy or loose slices. Set the firm slices on a rack to cool and harden, and place the flimsy slices back on the baking sheet and bake for another 10 minutes, being careful not to let the chips burn.

Continue baking in increments of 8–10 minutes until the chips have hardened. Allow them to cool on a rack.

Place the chips in a bowl, spray with coconut oil, and sprinkle with fresh ground rosemary and garlic.

Macronutrients/batch | 430 calories, 10g protein, 100g carbs, 0g fat, 15g fiber, 20g sugar

DAY 6
Delayed Gratification

DON'T GIVE UP

what you want most

for what you want now.

—Author Unknown

Instant gratification. Our lives are surrounded by the immediacy of social media, online shopping, and instant responses. The Internet never sleeps, after all. The result is that we never learn to delay because, well, we don't have to. Why should we when we can have it all and have it NOW!

The media and powerful market campaigns give us the impression that weight loss can be so simple and easy and in only weeks you'll see lasting results. The results of those fad diets that are so hard to stick to may seem wonderful, but how many people live a long and healthy life on a grapefruit diet? Or a pill. None.

Let me speak the simple truth that so many of us try so hard to deny: weight loss, fitness, and good health require the investment of time, wise food planning, and exercise. Don't sacrifice these for instant gratification.

Where are you giving way to instant gratification?

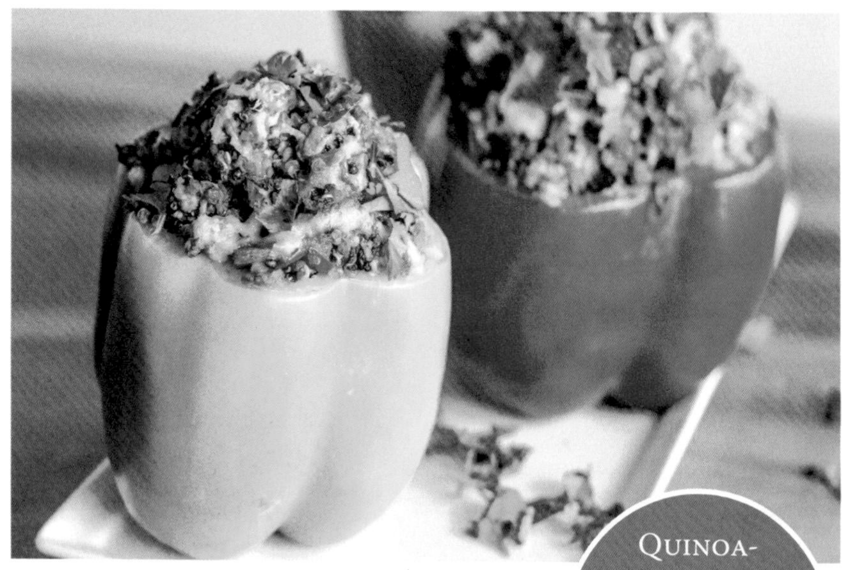

Quinoa-and-Chicken-Stuffed Bell Peppers

| 3 STUFFED PEPPERS |

Stuffed bell peppers are most definitely a healthy eating classic (at least in my book). This is one of my favorite meals that is protein packed, easy to customize (even for vegans), easy to prep, and family-approved!

Ingredients

1 lb extra lean ground chicken

1.5 cup cooked gluten-free quinoa

1/2 cup diced bell peppers

1.5 tbsp or 3 oz tomato paste

1 cup low sodium chicken broth

3 tbsp mozzarella

Seasonings for chicken:

smoked paprika, garlic, sea salt

For a vegan friendly version, use Portobello or tempeh, increase amount of quinoa, use veggie broth and cashew cheese

STEPS

Set the oven to 350°F.

In a pot, cook quinoa and set aside.

Season ground chicken and cook in a nonstick skillet.

When chicken is done cooking, add quinoa, tomato paste, diced bell peppers, chicken broth, and tomato paste. Mix and cook for 3 minutes on medium heat.

Cut the tops off 3 bell peppers and remove the inside. Place the mixture of chicken and quinoa in the bell peppers. Top with mozzarella.

Bake in the oven for about 20 minutes.

Smash them!

Macronutrients per pepper | 363 calories, 41g protein, 28g carbs, 9g fat

DAY 7
Have Fun

CREATIVITY IS

inventing, experimenting, growing, taking risks, breaking rules, making mistakes,

and having fun.

—Mary Lou Cook

One of the great joys of cooking is the creativity and experimenting, the mixing and the matching, the designing of the meals, and the joyful passion for mastering it as an art. I have found the making of food to awake all of my senses, touching my spirit, soul, and body. I feel alive in the kitchen.

What about you? Cooking may not be your thing, but what is? What are you doing to keep your life interesting and fun? You weren't created to merely do the same thing over and over until you feel like a zombie. Why just conform to what everyone else is doing? Break out of the rut and do something that even you might think is astounding. Start being daring and creative. Who says you don't have an invention inside you, or a book, or a green thumb? Stop being predictable; shake off the limits.

How can you unlock your creativity?

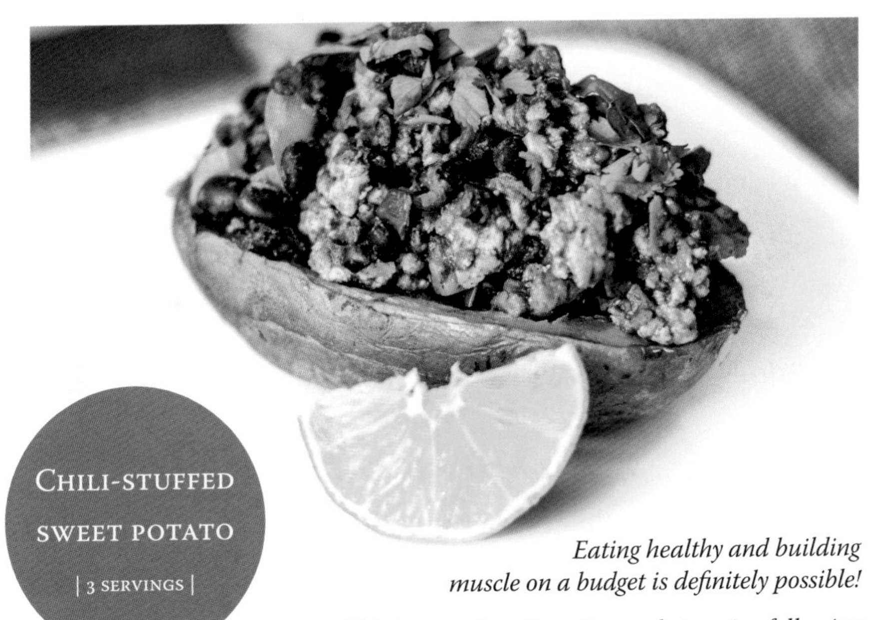

Chili-stuffed sweet potato

| 3 servings |

Eating healthy and building muscle on a budget is definitely possible!

This is one of my favorite meals to enjoy following a nice workout. It has a nice combination of sweet and savory flavors with high quality protein and complex carbohydrates to feed the muscles.

Ingredients

6 oz extra lean ground turkey

150g sweet potato (baked)

3/4 Roma tomato (diced)

1/8 cup low sodium black beans

1/8 cup green onions

Seasonings

1 tbsp McCormick low sodium chili seasoning, Mrs. Dash Chipotle seasoning (optional)

STEPS

Bake a sweet potato in the oven until soft.

Set a skillet on medium heat and add ground meat.

Chop the meat in the skillet with a spatula and add seasonings while it is cooking. When the meat is 70% finished, add tomatoes, green onions, and black beans. Mix together using a spatula.

Reduce the heat to low, cover the skillet, and cook for another 5–8 minutes.

When the sweet potato has finished baking, slice it in half, and scoop out just a little from the top to create a small hole.

Top the sweet potato with the chili mixture from the skillet.

Enjoy!

Approximate macronutrients | 381 calories, 47g protein, 41g carbs, 3g fats

WEEK 6 WRAP

1. What recipes did you try this week?

2. What did you like about the recipes?

3. What would you change next time?

4. What unique healthy meal did you create using one lean protein, one complex carbohydrate or power food, and one healthy fat?

5. How much have you progressed against your week 1 baseline?

6. What's your new, radical fitness goal?

» Weekly Challenge Checklist

Completed daily devotionals?	
Prepared 5 recipes from Week 1–6?	
Created your own healthy meal?	
Assessed your progress against week 1 baseline?	
Set a new radical fitness goal?	
Extra recipes created?	
Total challenges completed	

6-WEEK CHALLENGE WRAP-UP

Congrats! You've made it through the first 6 weeks of the rest of your life. . . . How do you feel?

....

What was your favorite part of the challenge?

....

What do you look forward to over the next 6 weeks? The next 6 months?

....

Who do you want to inspire to join this health and wellness journey with you?

....

Let's look back to see how you did...

Week 1 Challenge Points	
Week 2 Challenge Points	
Week 3 Challenge Points	
Week 4 Challenge Points	
Week 5 Challenge Points	
Week 6 Challenge Points	
Total Challenge Points	

So what's next? Time to encourage a friend or loved one to complete this 6-week challenge and see how you all stack up! Friendly competition can be a great way to support one another in your health and fitness journey. You can also continue to create unique and tasty meals with all of the knowledge you've acquired going through this 6-week transformation. Remember, this is a marathon, not a sprint! The new habits you've created will benefit you for the rest of your life. So keep it up and inspire someone else to do the same! Boom!

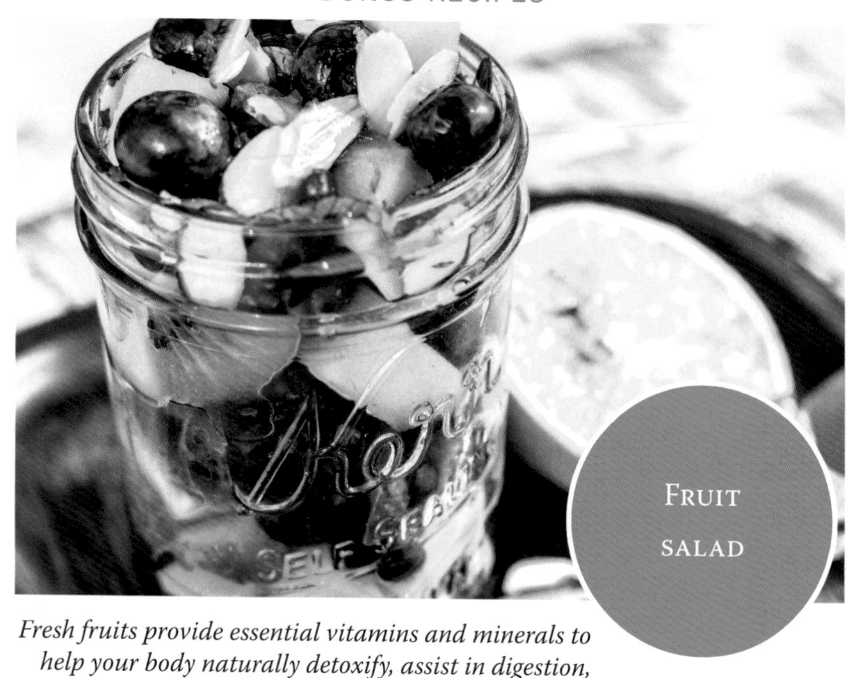

FRUIT SALAD

Fresh fruits provide essential vitamins and minerals to help your body naturally detoxify, assist in digestion, and help with the prevention of diseases.

Ingredients

- blueberries
- strawberries
- mango
- kiwi
- shaved almonds
- chopped mint
- drizzled with orange juice

Instead of shoveling out several dollars for simply one serving of a fruit salad at a restaurant, here are quick tips to make your next fruit salad "pop":

For one serving, use about 1/4 cup of 3–4 different fruits. I recommend using at least one berry (blueberry, blackberry, strawberry, raspberry) since berries are low-calorie yet provide a lot of flavor.

To increase the heartiness and boost the amount of protein and healthy carbohydrates, use almonds and/or granola.

Squeeze fresh orange (or other fruit) juice over the fruit salad, instead of honey or syrup, to add natural sweetness and flavor.

Garnish with herbs such as mint to increase the amount of fresh, robust flavors.

168 calories, 19g protein, 15g carbs, 4g fat, 3g fiber

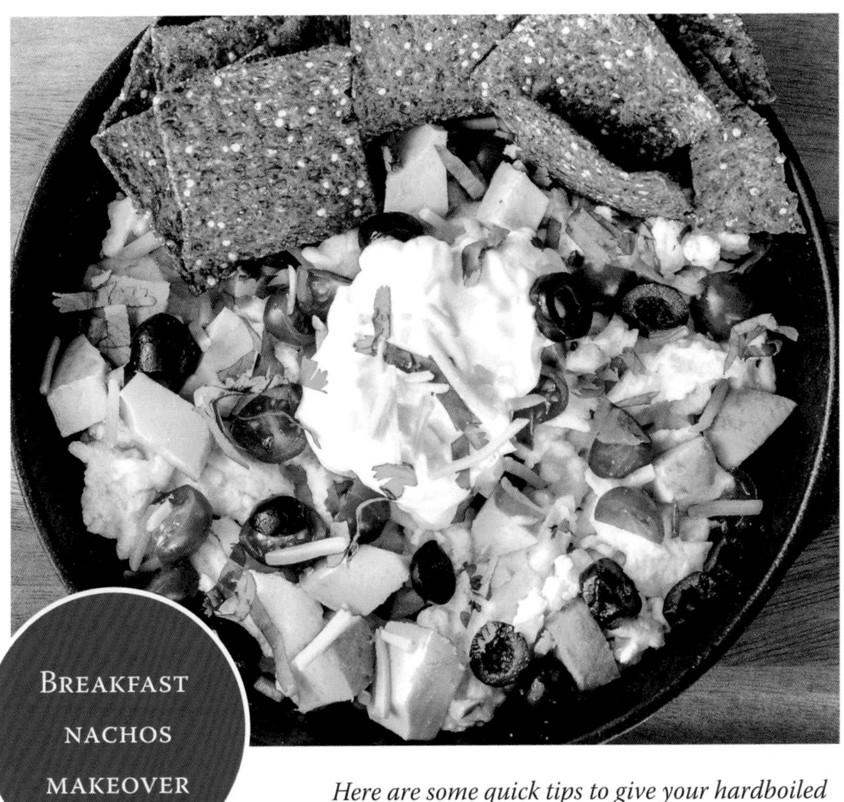

Breakfast nachos makeover

Break the rules of breakfast. It will make your new, healthy lifestyle more enjoyable and sustainable.

Here are some quick tips to give your hardboiled egg whites and oatmeal breakfast meal a fresh, vibrant makeover:

Scramble egg whites and season to taste with garlic, sea salt, cumin, and pepper.

Use blue corn, wheat, or whole grain tortillas or chips instead of eating oatmeal.

Add some heart healthy fat by adding a few chopped pieces of avocado and, if you like, some black olives.

Top with 1 tablespoon of Greek yogurt instead of sour cream.

Sprinkle with cilantro for added flavor, and if you're feeling adventurous, 1 tablespoon of mozzarella or reduced fat cheddar cheese.

And BOOM!

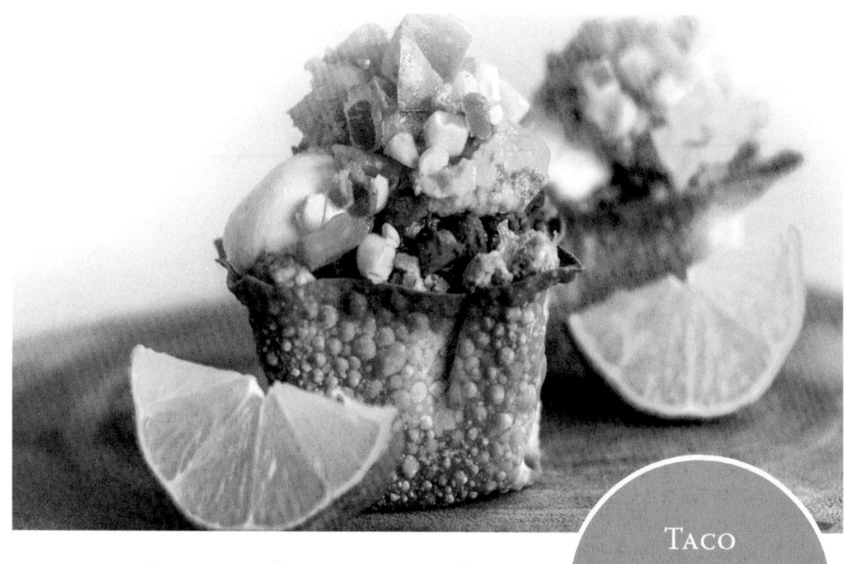

Taco cups

| 12 taco cups |

Just in time for your next watch party or for a family of picky eaters! Try these loaded taco cups that everyone will enjoy.

Ingredients

1–2 lbs extra lean turkey meat

15 oz can low sodium black beans

1/2 onion diced

2 tbsp of garlic paste

1/2 cup Greek yogurt

1/2 cup guacamole

1/4 cup steamed corn

1/3 cup pico de gallo

12 egg roll wraps (Nasoya brand)

Seasonings

coconut aminos, onions, Mrs. Dash

STEPS

Preheat oven to 360°F.

Spray muffin pan with coconut oil.

Fill pan with the desired number of egg roll wraps. Place the wrap in the muffin hole and form cup. Trim the edges of each of the wraps.

Bake wraps for 12 minutes at 360°F. Remove and let cool.

Season ground turkey. Add 1 tbsp of garlic paste and 1/4 of the diced onions.

Cook in a nonstick skillet on medium-high heat until done. Set aside.

In a separate skillet, sauté the remainder of the diced onions with 1 tbsp of garlic paste.

Add black beans to the skillet. Mash the black beans with a spatula to create a paste. Cover and cook on low heat for 10 minutes.

Time to load your taco cups. Fill each cup with 1–2 oz ground turkey, then 1 tbsp of the black bean paste, 1/2 tbsp of Greek yogurt, 1/2 tbsp of guacamole, 1 tsp of steamed corn, and finally 1 tsp of pico de gallo.

Macronutrients per taco cup | 188 calories, 18g protein, 19g carbs, 3g fat

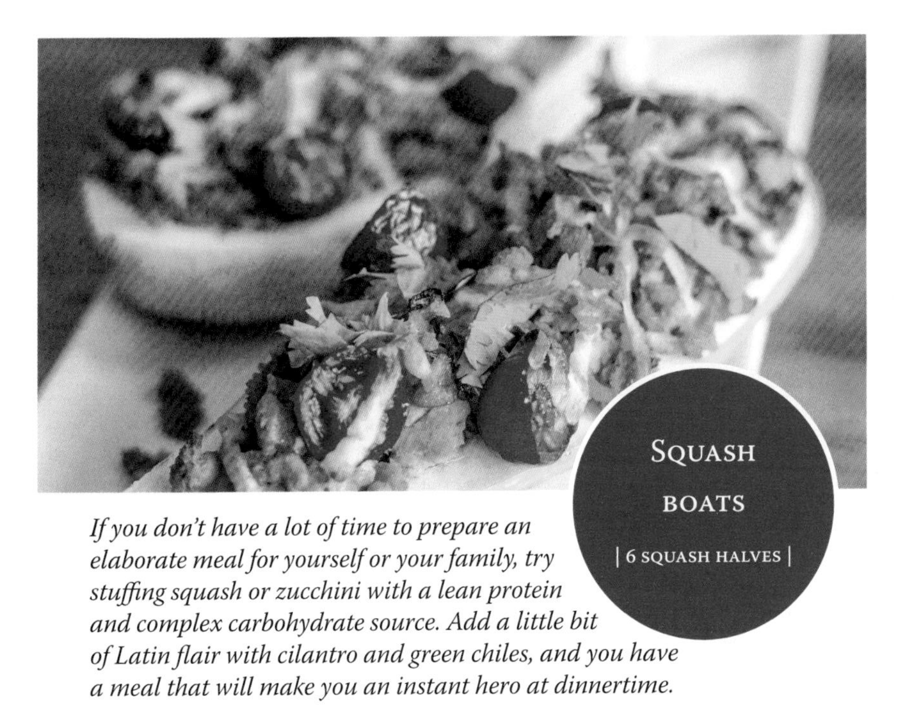

Squash boats

| 6 squash halves |

If you don't have a lot of time to prepare an elaborate meal for yourself or your family, try stuffing squash or zucchini with a lean protein and complex carbohydrate source. Add a little bit of Latin flair with cilantro and green chiles, and you have a meal that will make you an instant hero at dinnertime.

Ingredients

1 lb lean ground chicken

4 oz hatch green chiles (mild, canned)

1 cup cooked brown and wild rice mix

1 tbsp garlic paste

10 cherry tomatoes (sliced in half)

1/2 tbsp cumin

3 tbsp reduced fat mozzarella (optional)

Fresh cilantro (chopped)

STEPS

Set oven to 405°F.

Slice yellow squash in half and carve out part of the insides with the seeds.

Set a nonstick skillet on medium-high heat. Add garlic paste and ground chicken, then cumin seasoning, and cook until chicken is 70% finished. Break up the chicken with a wooden spatula so that it does not bind together.

Toss in green chiles and cooked rice. Mix together and cook until the chicken is 90% finished.

Place the squash halves on a baking sheet.

Fill the squash with the chicken and chile mixture.

Slice cherry tomatoes in half and place on top of the meat mixture.

Top with mozzarella cheese, about 1/2 tbsp for each boat half.

Bake for 20 minutes for cooked yet firm squash.

Remove and top with fresh cilantro.

Macronutrients per squash halves | 168 calories, 19g protein, 15g carbs, 4g fat, 3g fiber

SUPER FOODS AND COMPLEX CARBOHYDRATES

These are some of my favorite foods that are packed with nutrients and vitamins to give me the energy to power through the day and any intense workout. Also, these are my go-to complex carbohydrates that I enjoy incorporating into my diet on a regular basis—there are tons out there, but "when in doubt," I go back to this list for inspiration.

Super foods

- Asparagus
- Avocados
- Beets
- Berries: blueberries, raspberries, blackberries, strawberries
- Broccoli
- Colorful bell peppers
- Cacao or dark chocolate
- Coconut oil (for cooking)
- Greek yogurt
- Kale
- Kiwi
- Spinach
- Zucchini

Complex carbohydrates

- Freekeh
- Oatmeal
- Plantains
- Quinoa
- Sweet potatoes

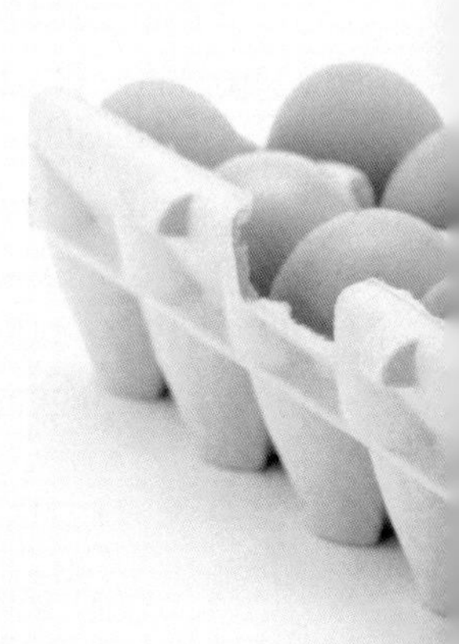

PROTEIN SOURCES

Here are some of my favorite protein sources that I enjoy incorporating into recipes and meals. Keep in mind that while they may be proven sources of protein, they vary in terms of the amount of fat and even carbohydrates with the vegetarian options. If you are following a medically prescribed diet that is low in fat, be sure to check the amount of fat per serving.

Animal sources	Eggs Bison (lean) Chicken breast (boneless, skinless) Flank steak (lean) Ground turkey (lean) Salmon White fish Cottage cheese Greek yogurt Goat cheese
Vegetarian sources	Tempeh Black beans Green peas Quinoa Ezekiel bread Hummus Nuts and seeds

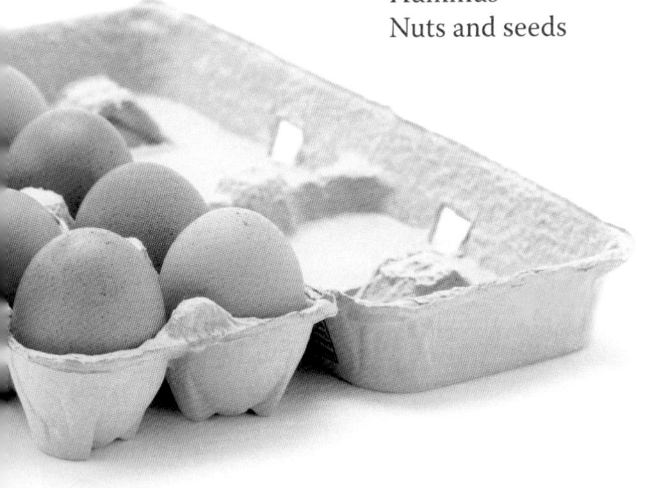

SAMPLE GROCERY LIST

Preparing some of your meals in advance is a proven way to ensure you maintain a healthy diet and make healthier food choices throughout the week. Here's a sample grocery list that I've used here in Texas that ran me about $120 for at least 5 meals per day for 5 days.

Protein
72 oz (~4.5 lbs) chicken breast
40 oz (~2.5 lbs) white fish
35 oz (~2.25 lbs) lean flank steak
2 cartons eggs
2 cartons egg whites

Carbohydrates
3 bags brown rice bags
1 carton instant oatmeal
1 box quinoa
2 large sweet potatoes

Produce
2 medium avocados
1 small carton blueberries
1 carton strawberries
2 bundles asparagus
1 box spinach
3 cucumbers
4 lemons
3 bell peppers
small carton fresh pico de gallo

Fats
Natural nut butter

Dairy
carton almond milk (this is not dairy but found in dairy section)
small carton goat cheese
small carton cottage cheese
8 oz Greek yogurt 2%

GETTING FLAVOR IN YOUR DIET

Finding ways to enhance your meals with seasonings can be a little overwhelming if you're just starting out. I remember going to the seasoning aisle and just staring at it hoping someone would come along and give me a recommendation. Here are the spices, seasonings, and sauces that I always have on hand to toss into a recipe.

Seasonings
- paprika
- cumin
- cayenne pepper
- turmeric
- ginger (powder)
- coriander
- curry powder
- garlic powder
- onion powder
- Mrs. Dash no sodium seasonings
- sea salt
- Bragg's Liquid Aminos
- pepper

Sauces
- natural, organic BBQ sauce
- Sriracha
- Dijon mustard
- Red chili pepper paste

Spices
- cinnamon
- nutmeg
- allspice
- vanilla extract

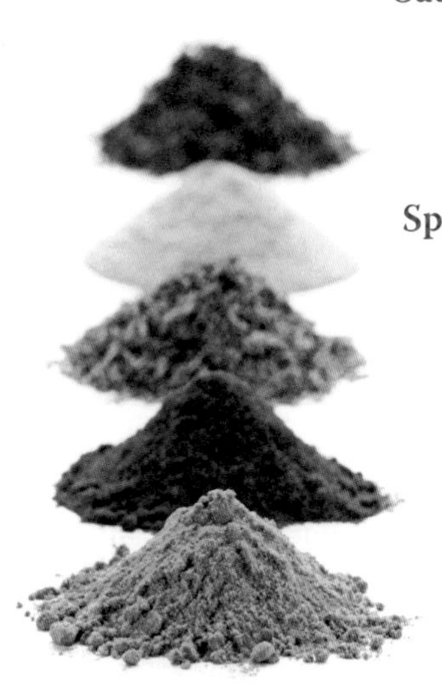

5 HEALTHY TIPS TO ENRICH YOUR JOURNEY

1 *Hydrate by Drinking Mostly Pure Water.* Most people tend to overlook the importance of drinking adequate amounts of water or non-sugary beverages daily. Fluids such as water help to transport and distribute nutrients from the foods you consume throughout your entire body. Aim to drink between 10 to 12 cups daily, and more if you are active to account for the amount of fluid you lose during strenuous activity, such as exercise.

2 *Get Educated.* Spend time reading material from reputable sources about the nutritional value of the foods you choose to eat. One of the best decisions I ever made was walking into that bookstore and purchasing a variety of materials about nutrition to get different perspectives so I could make the best decision for my goals and my body.

3 *Practice Self-Control.* Eat only until you are satisfied and not until you are full. This may take some time mastering, but it is largely important for portion control and healthy living. There is nothing wrong with saving food and finishing it later. If you are a competitor or athlete, well, you may need to "stuff your face" with your carefully measured portion of food in order to meet your caloric requirement for the day. But for most, eating until you are satisfied is a healthy practice. And remember, there is a difference between being hungry versus being thirsty; so before you get the urge to eat, drink a glass of water first—you may not feel hungry afterward.

4 *Have It Your Way.* Enjoying a night out with friends and family does not have to derail your commitment to making wiser, healthy choices. Don't be afraid to be specific when asking your server about what a particular dish contains or how it is prepared. Customize your meal and swap out food items so that you can stay as close as possible to your plan. I generally like to stick with grilled chicken breast and grilled seafood when eating out at restaurants.

5 *Be Consistent.* I enjoy eating several small meals throughout the day to give my body time to process the food I eat. Remember, everyone's body is different, and some people have experienced positive results by eating only 3 times per day. For me, that meant going longer periods of time without eating, thereby causing me to overeat at those 3 meals because I was extremely hungry. When I made the switch to eating continuously throughout the day, I avoided that problem. At the end of the day, this is a lifestyle, and you should do what works best for you.